Eat More

A Handbook for Real Health

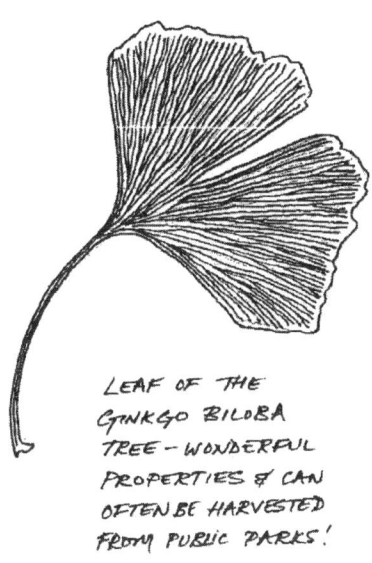

LEAF OF THE
GINKGO BILOBA
TREE - WONDERFUL
PROPERTIES & CAN
OFTEN BE HARVESTED
FROM PUBLIC PARKS!

by Steve Charter

(the illustrations too)

Published in the UK by:

Steve Charter

The rights of Steve Charter to be identified as author of this work has been asserted by him in accordance with the Copyright, Designs and Patents Act 1988.

Text copyright © 2016 Steve Charter. All rights reserved.

Fully revised edition Eat More Raw Too published 2016, by Steve Charter

First edition (Eat More Raw) published 2004, by Permanent Publications

All rights reserved. No part of this publication may be reproduced, stored in a retrieval system, rebound or transmitted in any form or by any means, electronic, mechanical, photocopying, recording or otherwise, without the prior permission of the author.

Acknowledgements

I express great thanks to Robert Hart (1913-2000) for encouraging me to write this book, and for his contribution to it; Tony Wright for his helpful comments on the various drafts, for introducing me to the raw lifestyle back in 1994, for writing *Return to the Brain of Eden* (with Graham Gynn, Inner Traditions), and for the extraordinary insights contained therein; Morgan for that Permaculture Course back in '94, for being Morgan and for creating Turners Field; to all those who have made direct contributions to this book, and to those that have contributed indirectly; to all of those involved in PFAF over the years; Sure/Liefde/Kerry Martin of Tiaia and her many 'cellves'; Aranya for all his permaculture teaching and for being a living, loving example of the paradise garden way – and for his Foreword to this book; to all my Ecoforest friends, those that made it happen, and those that made it what it was by being there for however long they stayed; to all those that have helped develop the raw foods movement, including the early pioneers that are no longer with us and to those that are doing it now; Martin Crawford for the important and inspiring work of the Agroforestry Research Trust; so many authors, teachers and raw food and permaculture activists, past, present and future, all of whom are part of the positive and peaceful (r)evolution towards health and sustainability of which this book is a part; Bill Mollison and David Holmgren for sowing the seeds and doing the 'educational mulching' that started permaculture off, and the positive, inspiring, solutions-oriented permaculture movement in the UK and around the world; Nichol Clarke for helping revitalizing the context for *Eat More Raw Too*; and a huge 'thank you' to Maddy and Tim Harland, John Adams, Tony Rollinson and the rest of the team at Permanent Publications for their unstintingly positive and supportively critical comments on the first edition of this book and their support in getting this 2nd edition out, even though they decided not to publish it themselves in the end! Thank you all.

And for this Second Edition, love and thanks to John and Michael, though you may not realise it, one way or another you've really helped me make many positive changes in this second edition of this book, so I hope it's a book that may help you sometime too, if or when you need it.

Steve Charter

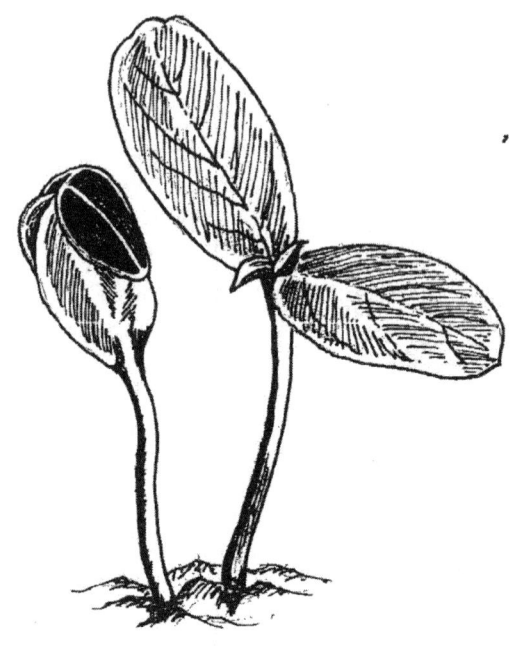

Sunflower greens – *yum!*

CONTENTS

Foreword to Eat More Raw Too 11
Foreword to Eat More Raw 12
PART 1: Introduction 13
    Raw Foods – Fad or Feeling? 15
    Sustainability and Health – Fad or Future? 19
        Why Raw Food and Sustainability? 22
PART 2: The Problem – Ill Health is Natural 24
    Acceptance or Response–Ability? 24
    Personal and Planetary Health 24
    Institutional Science v's the Blatantly Flipping Obvious 27
    Health and Sustainability - Where Are We Heading? 33
    Life in the 21st Century 34
    A Positive Vision 35
    Creating Real Health 36
PART 3: The Solution – Health Is Natural 37
    Interconnectedness 37
    Working With Nature: A Practical Philosophy For Sustainable & Healthy Living 37
        Brief Interlude: If It's Good Enough For Gandhi 39
Working With Nature: The Route to Personal & Planetary Health 41
    The Big Challenge to Us as Individuals and the World 43
        The Creative Margins 43
        The Stuck and Stagnant Mainstream 43
PART 4: The Strategy - Thrive by Meeting Your Needs 44
    Sustainable Living Means Meeting Your Healthy Needs 44
    Real Health 47
    Knowledge as the Fruit of Extended Observation & Experience 48
    Nature as Your Guide to Health 50
    Sustainable Living, Health and Permaculture 53
    Earth Care: Ecological Sustainability 54
    People Care: Meeting Human Needs 55
    Fair Share: Equity in Choice, and Sharing Surplus 55
    Attitude Principles and Their Benefits to Diet and Health 56
        Work With Nature, Not Against It 56
        Everything Gardens (or Everything Has Effects) 58
        Maximum Output for Minimum Effort 60

Yield is (Theoretically) Unlimited...62
The Problem is the Solution 62
Harvest Only Sunshine (or Closing the Loop) 64
Some 'Frequently Asked Questions' About Raw Foods 66
The Cooking Question 66
The Protein Question 67
The Fat Question 68
The Meat Question...70
The Starch and Carbohydrate Question 72
The Nutritional & Health Research Question 73
Frequent and Less Common Questions and Answers 76
PART 5: The Action Plan - The Practicalities...77
Transitional Living 77
Practical Actions 81
Making the Transition 82
Detoxification and Cleansing: a natural process 85
Other Issues: Climatic, Seasonal and Local Foods 88
Minerals and Cleansing 88
Acid / Alkaline Balance 89
Sodium / Potassium Balance 90
Take Care of Yourself in the Short & Long Term: Maintaining Balance 91
Chronic Illnesses and Major Health Challenges 94
The *Eat More Raw* Path As A Spiritual Journey..95
An Eastern Spiritual Perspective 96
Eat More Raw Parenting – before and after birth 101
F.A.Q's About The Practicalities of Eating More Raw 105
FAQ1 - How do I go to roughly 50% raw, 50% cooked? 105
FAQ2 - Will the food be satisfying enough? 105
FAQ3 - What is a typical diet for a week? 106
FAQ4 - What do I do about sourcing all the ingredients...? 107
FAQ5 - How do you stop a raw diet/lifestyle becoming boring?.....................108
FAQ6 - What's the ideal raw diet?..109
FAQ7 - What extra equipment would I need? Is a juicer essential?................109
FAQ8 - What are the best things to sprout? 110
FAQ9 - What do you eat when you're out, or visiting friends or family? 111
What are the best things to drink and how important are they? 113
Let's Be Honest, Are there any dangers? 114

    So what actually is your position on raw foods? 117
    12 Reasons to Eat More Raw...119
    Making The Transition Easier and More Social 119
PART 6: Designing Real Health 120
    The Twelve Petalled Flower of Health 120
        Meditation..124
        Positive Mental and Spiritual Nutrition..125
        Programme Yourself With Positivity, Health and Sustainability 127
    A 6 Month to 1 Year Outline Plan 128
    Use These Tools To Help You 129
PART 7: The Role of Permaculture 130
    The Idea And Practice of Creating Many Benefits 131
    Learning About Permaculture: The Ethics and Design Principles 131
    Permaculture Design Tools and Strategies 133
        Zones..134
        Bioregional Zoning...136
        Sectors 138
        Slopes 138
        Permaculture Techniques..139
        Forest Gardening...140
        Useful Plants and Plant Typologies 143
        Flowering Plants, and The Role of Flowers and Bees 144
        Wild Foods...145
        Other Useful Plants 146
    The Design Process..146
        The OBREDIM Design Process 147
        Your Permaculture Toolbag...148
    Your Health and Sustainability Pathway 149
        Growing and Buying Foods to Cook 149
        Useful Resources 150
PART 8: There's Lots of Information & Inspiration Out There 152
    Section One: Lifestyles, Landscapes and Philosophies of Living 152
        The Forest Garden Diet, Lifestyle and Philosophy, by *Robert A de J Hart*........152
        Indoor Gardening and Living Foods, by Elaine Bruce 153
        Paradise Gardening, by Joe Hollis...155
        Free and Natural Life: On the Trail of Simplicity and Love, by Sibila 157
        Plants for a Future and The Agroforestry Research Trust 159

Section Two: Examples of Major Healing & Personal Change 160
  Jatinda Daniels: cured severe arthritis 160
  Angela Stokes: achieved significant, sustained and weight-loss. 160
  Dave Klein: cured his Ulcerative Colitis 163
  Shazzie: overcame depression, lethargy, brain-fog & created a life she loves 164
PART 9: The Conclusion 166
  This Is The Beginning Not The End... 166
  Shift From Consuming Life to Producing Health 168
PART 10: Recipes, Food Preparation and Meal Ideas 169
  Steve's Recipe for Success 169
  Some Really Delicious and Radically Healthy Recipes 170
    Breakfast and Morning 171
    Other simple snack lunch options 172
  Savoury Dishes From Around The World 173
    Three Oriental Dishes 173
    Three Middle Eastern Dishes 174
    Three Curry Dishes 176
    Three Mexican and South American Dishes 177
    Two Italian Dishes 177
    Other Dishes 178
    Raw Soups 179
    Sundried (in a warm climate) or Dehydrator Dishes 180
    A Culinary Tip – two versions of 'The 5 Tastes' 180
    Other Savoury Dishes for Anywhere and Everywhere 180
    Some Other Staples and Great Salad Dishes 181
    A Different Kind of Recipe for Salad Success 182
  Sweet Dishes 182
    A Cautionary Note On Raw Sweets and Puddings 184
  Some healthy options for a 'mainly raw' lifestyle 185
    Breakfast 185
    Practical Working Lunch or School Lunch 185
    Dinner 185
PART 11: The Appendices 186
  Appendix 1: About The Author 186
  Appendix 2: Contacts, Resources and Information 191
    Raw Food and Natural Health Contacts and Information 191
    Other Living/Raw Food Reading 192

- Raw Recipe Books ... 193
- Raw Parenting Resources ... 193
- Permaculture Information, Networks and Organisations ... 194
  - Australia: ... 195
  - Excellent Temperate Climate Resources *(e.g. for Europe and N America)* ... 195
  - Permaculture Websites ... 195
  - Publishers and Mail Order Book Suppliers ... 195
  - Permaculture Reading ... 196
  - Seed and Plant Suppliers ... 197
  - The Food System, Economy, Sustainability & The Medical System ... 197
- Appendix 3: An Outline for Establishing a Forest Garden ... 198
  - Temperate Climates ... 198
  - Sub-Tropical and Mediterranean Type Climates ... 202
- Index ... 204
- Other Books by Steve Charter: ... 204

FOREWORD TO EAT MORE RAW TOO

I've had the great pleasure of knowing Steve for almost two decades now, meeting him first at a small UK raw food gathering back when such ideas were less popular. Soon afterwards I moved into a shared house on the outskirts of Exeter, appropriately named 'Hales', a place already home to Steve and several other raw food eaters. Back then the FRESH network magazine was being run from the house and my subsequent involvement with that and sharing meals together taught me a lot about the value of raw foods. I made some great friends too.

My main work for the last decade or so has been in teaching permaculture. Steve was responsible for that too. As part of his teaching apprenticeship he organised for a two-week permaculture design course to take place in our home. I signed up and the rest is history.

After Hales I moved to Eire and Steve made his way to southern Spain where for ten years he had a key role in running a raw food land based project called Ecoforest. During that time we visited each other and despite being several years older than me, whenever I met him I always thought how young he looked.

All the time I've known him, Steve has written down his thoughts and experiences, publishing a number of different booklets and papers, culminating in the first edition of *Eat More Raw* back in 2004. This latest edition adds Steve's many thoughts from the ten years since. It weaves the seemingly separate worlds of healthy living, raw food and permaculture together into a cohesive whole. Permaculture encourages us, indeed urges us to pay attention to the natural world, to learn what makes her healthy and successful and to apply those same strategies to meeting our needs in the modern world. The raw food doctrine says that cooking is unnatural. Neither movement seems to have the full picture. Standing with a foot in both worlds, Steve weaves them together, showing that they are two sides of the same thing.

Eat More Raw Too is a book at the leading edge of its cross-disciplinary field. Whether you have come to it from permaculture, from healthy living and raw foods, or from neither, there is much to learn here, the kind of learning that can change your life. That's certainly been the case for me.

Steve has always been a pioneer, a forward thinker, and in my mind someone well worth listening to. Here in your hands you have a chance to catch up with him for a moment, and speaking from my own fortunate experience, I advise you to dive in!

Aranya - Permaculture teacher and teacher of teachers, designer, author of Permaculture Design: a step-by-step guide, *diploma tutor, film maker, creator of Permaculture Musicians project and producer of* Earth Stars CD, *website designer, innovator, barefoot runner, singer, member of Designed Visions permaculture cooperative and much more. Oh, and a very good friend, to me and many other fortunate folk!*

For more information on Aranya's work see: http://www.learnpermaculture.com/

FOREWORD TO EAT MORE RAW

Progress tends to come in spurts. Like the well-known plateaus that people experience in their personal training, all of our learning is subject to periods of hibernation. It takes time to get used to new levels of performance, advances in technology, linguistic nuances, social progress. Once we get used to the new way and gain some experience in using it, better ways become apparent. Such is growth. That is what this book is all about; bringing the reader to a new found level of awareness.

Specialization is a strong indicator of growth. In the raw food movement, there have been vast waves of specialization in the past few years. Each new aspect of this specialization has raised the awareness of those involved in the movement. This made it easier for people to succeed as raw fooders, or to better perform their outreach or educational missions.

Specialization has helped those already in the movement, but it has not really resulted in growth of the movement. For growth to occur, a bigger overall picture must be observed and put into effect. That, exactly, is what you will find within these pages; a profoundly new perspective that beautifully merges many varied aspects of the healthful lifestyle.

Let me use the sport of golf as an example, for a moment. Golf is an extremely challenging game to play. It is comprised of many aspects. The number of variables are huge. You may get better and better at one aspect of the game but see no indicator of such by an overall lowering of your total end score. Practise as you may, golf can remain extremely frustrating, especially if you are attached to the score as an indicator of how well you played the game. Then, one day, things come together in a new way. The bits and pieces begin to fall into place. After a few holes, your entire perception of yourself and the game begins to change. A new self confidence arises. You can even express your performance with a vocabulary that until today had eluded you. Lo and behold, at game's end, several strokes have come off of your all time low score. You have evolved.

This book marks the beginning of a new era. It marks the culmination of many years of cultural, environmental, and food style advances. It marks a union of diverse areas of study. Within these pages, what were until now separate and distinct fields of endeavour have come together. They have been artistically united in a fashion that will bring the reader to new found understandings of a bigger picture of healthful living.

We stand on the precipice of survival. We can choose to continue doing what we have always done in the past, in which case the demise of the human race is predictable. We can instead move forward, experiment, and make lifestyle modifications. Armed with better information, humans tend to make better decisions. I believe that reading this book will leave you better informed, make you a better person, and give you many of the tools that you need to emerge from the cultural cocoon as the butterfly that we all wish to become.

Dr Douglas N. Graham *(President of Healthful Living International)*

PART 1: Introduction

There is a lot more to food than meets the eye.

Our food can be a vehicle for positive personal and planetary change, and for creating health. Alternatively, it can create and sustain ill-health, economic exploitation and ecological damage. Food and the way we obtain it is connected to a whole network of different effects, chain reactions and chains of responsibility in our lives and in the world we are part of. Food affects and is affected by activities in the economy, society and the web of life – the outside world. Food is also affected by and affects our internal world – our mind, body, spirit and emotions. And vice versa.

This book offers guidance on what happens when we eat *more* raw foods – specifically fresh and organic:
- fruits
- vegetables and salads
- nuts and seeds
- sprouted pulses and grains
- raw superfoods and 'food-state' / raw supplements
- cold pressed oils, seaweeds, herbs and so on

This is a book about:
- eating more raw food
- the possibilities of eating around 50% raw foods or all raw, for short or long periods
- the effects in your life when you eat more raw foods
- the effects in the wider world when you eat more raw foods
- the effects of growing more of the food that you eat, or at least some of it

So it's a book that is relevant to you if you:
- eat no raw foods at all, eat 100% rawfoods, or anywhere in between
- are a meat eater, a vegan or a vegetarian
- are a chocoholic or junk food addict
- are a wholefoods fanatic
- grow all of your own food... or none of it

This is a book for people who ask questions about:
- the health of their body, mind and spirit
- the health of their family and friends
- the health of humanity as a whole and its effects on this extraordinary planet we live on
- the health of the abundant, varied yet utterly interconnected and evolving eco-systems on which we and all life on the planet depend.

It's a book about the effects of what we eat on ourselves and on the world in which we live.

So if you care about your own health and the health of children, friends or relatives, about the health of your home, planet earth, what we are doing now, and how that is affecting our culture and other cultures, the planet and all life on it, then this is a book that you need to read.

This book shows how you can use the food you eat and the cause-and-effect-relationships that are connected to it to inspire, encourage and accelerate positive change. In particular this book suggests that by working with nature, we can significantly improve the health of people and planet – and create a *personal culture of health* and a wider *culture of health*, within a wider *culture of change*.

This book is relevant for people interested in ethical living, sustainable ways of living, social and global food issues and the relationship between health and nutrition. And it's a book for people who are seeking a simple, natural, straight-forward perspective on health and nutrition – which is so different from the industrial, profit-oriented and medicinal-drug based view of chronic illness, disease and food that dominates our society in the early 21_{st} century.

If you want to change the inner and outer effects of your life, and be part of a positive culture of change, then this is a book for you.

So what's in this book, then?

Overall the book is *three books in one*: a) a practical guide to 'eating more raw', b) a guide to designing and creating real health, and c) the first book to apply permaculture to health, in terms of growing more of your own food and how *applying permaculture design principles, tools and practices to the field of health, leads naturally to certain healthy conclusions*.

This first part of the book (Parts 1 & 2) explores and exposes the nature of health and sustainability 'problems' (a negative interpretation) – or if you prefer, 'issues' (a neutral interpretation) or 'opportunities', which is the positive interpretation. It sets out the basic principles that will help you to understand the cause-and-effect nature of these problems, issues and opportunities. There are a few points about our culture and its relationship to health that need hammering home - so that is done in this first section, and I recommend you stick with it.

The second part of the book (Parts 3 & 4, from p.37), and most of the book in fact, covers the practical 'solutions' to the 'problems' - the positive, creative responses that directly improve our health and increase our sustainability, covering the strategies and, in Part 5, *The Practicalities* of improving health and adopting *a health creating diet and lifestyle*. In Parts 6 & 7 we look at *how to design real health* (and the role of permaculture in this), to help you see that you can produce at least some of your own healthy and affordable food very easily, whether you have a garden or not, and to provide you with practical attitudes, tools and ways of thinking that are relevant to your lifestyle as a whole, what you eat and the environmental impacts of your life.

The next section (Part 8) includes some inspirational offerings from wise and experienced friends and personal stories from people who have overcome really significant health challenges, covering many aspects of the eat more raw lifestyle: people's journeys of change and deepened understanding. The final Parts 9 & 10 of the book include brief conclusions and then a detailed practical guide to preparing a good and tasty variety of raw meals, with a great range of delicious and *practical day-to-day raw recipes* and handy hints, followed by a selection of really useful information in the Appendices section on raw food, natural health and permaculture. Which all sounds like quite a feast of information and inspiration to me, so I hope it does to you too!

Raw Foods – Fad or Feeling?

Most importantly this book will help you understand the natural basis of health. It also helps you understand what happens when we eat more raw foods, for short or longer periods of time, and shows how we can grow more of these foods ourselves, individually and as a culture.

These ideas were new to me when I first heard of them, but I listened and then I tried them – and once I tried them for myself I found that in fact they felt good and made a lot of sense. So let's be clear: whilst it is still unusual to eat mainly or only raw foods, it is not actually weird at all – it's just unfamiliar for most of us. The idea may be new to your mind – I found that the reality was that it felt utterly natural to my body.

So is eating more raw foods or eating mainly raw foods (fruit, veg, seed sprouts, nuts, dried fruit, fresh juice, etc.) a fad? Yes, certainly for some people it is. But emphatically 'No' it is not for the vast majority that try it, and continue with it. And if you want to know why, then all is revealed within the pages of this book!

In fact eating mainly (i.e. 50%+ of your diet) or only raw foods is highly recommended by a variety of notable people. Robert Hart, who was an inspiration to many in the British and worldwide organic and permaculture movements, recommended a minimum 70% raw diet.[1] Robert drew his ideas from Mahatma Gandhi, who followed the principles of natural hygiene and ate a mainly raw diet for many years, seeing a simple natural diet as a vital part of his spiritual and political life. Interestingly, coming from a very different perspective, American success 'guru' Anthony Robbins recommends a very similar 70% raw diet in his book *Unlimited Power* because he sees vibrant health as essential for being successful in life, whilst the Australian fast bowling test cricketer Peter Siddle consumes 20 bananas a day as part of his high fruit and veg vegan diet, giving him excellent stamina and faster recovery times.

So people get into raw food for a number of reasons. Some people try it as a health experiment, perhaps having tried macrobiotics or the Hay Diet before. In fact the raw lifestyle has been popular in Hollywood and California, with actors Demi Moore and Woody Harrelson being some of the long-standing celebrity pioneers, joined along the way by Alicia Silverstone, Angela Basset, supermodel Carol Alt and possibly Sting, according to some sources. However, my guess is that the famous people who've stuck to the lifestyle are like anyone else, in that they have generally made this choice for reasons that are much stronger than mere fashion.

Some people see a difference in a friend or relation, whilst others may be given or chance upon a book, CD or DVD, or go to a talk or seminar, that opens their eyes to a whole new world they were not aware of before. In contrast, some start eating more raw foods by following their intuition, simplifying their diet and listening carefully to their body's deeper needs and desires. With a cleaner diet it becomes easier and easier to hear the body's sense of the foods that feel really good. This form of intuitive eating, is described by Sibila later in this book (and in her own books in Spanish), and in more detail in *Feel Good Food* by Susie Miller and Karen Knowler.[2]

---

[1] Robert Hart, *Forest Gardening*, Green Books (2001).

[2] The Women's Press, London (2000).

Others discover raw foods on a search for a more ethical, sustainable or spiritual way of living, feeling it to be a compassionate way of life, and a natural extension of vegetarianism or veganism, or being 'green'. With an interest in its spiritual benefits, some follow the tradition of eating mainly raw fruit amongst gurus in India, or find powerful references in ancient texts, including the *Bhagavad-Gita*, the *Bible*[3] and in *The Essene Gospels*[4]. Others see its numerous ecological benefits.

However, the majority come to raw foods by understanding its benefits in achieving improved health and fitness. Some are already relatively healthy and are seeking an even healthier lifestyle. And as a perfect example of this, the tennis player Martina Navratilova – possibly the most successful sports woman of all time – by eating plant based natural foods, with a good percentage of juicing and raw foods in her diet, as part of her total fitness regime, was able to maintain supreme levels of both physical and mental fitness late in her career, way after the age at which most athletes start to decline[5].

At a different end of the spectrum, when we come to the major health challenges of obesity and food disorders, Angela Stokes' inspiring writings and website (www.rawreform.com) show how significant, sustained and healthy weight loss can be a huge draw for others – more on this later. Meanwhile, many other people arrive at raw foods through a chronic illness, having heard or read about how raw food has greatly helped a healing process to take place in others – the movie *Fat, Sick and Nearly Dead* provides one such example. Raw foods, particularly green juices and 'living foods' (see Elaine Bruce's section later) have helped many people to fight and reduce the impacts of frightening chronic conditions or 'lifestyle diseases' such as cancer, heart-disease, diabetes, candida, colitis and obesity related conditions, and have significantly improved quality of life for people with severe arthritis, asthma or eczema.

In any situation, the most powerful healing and health creating effects will be felt by adopting a multi-tactic approach, ideally with exercise, meditation, and other lifestyle changes – changing the external conditions that helped create the chronic illness, and working on the internal conditions to enable healing to take place. Alongside switching to mainly raw foods, meditating, doing yoga and using various therapies, I've heard of people stopping watching TV and buying a wide selection of comedy videos to seriously use laughter to fight cancer.[6]

A large number of people explore the *eat more raw* lifestyle with an awareness of several of these issues, creating various benefits in their life from making one key change, suggesting the appealing idea that well informed choices can help us eat our way towards health and sustainability.

---

[3] Genesis 1.29 states: *And God said, Behold I have given you every herb bearing seed, which is upon the face of all the earth, and every tree, in which is the fruit of a tree yielding seed; to you it shall be for meat.*

[4] The Essene Gospels of Peace, *The Original Hebrew and Aramaic Texts, translated and edited by Edmond Bordeaux Szekely, International Biogenic Society*

[5] See her talk on Youtube: ***Martina Navratilova: Plant-Based Diet Is Best***

[6] The film *Patch Adams* starring Robin Williams, and the book it is based on, presents one perhaps valuable perspective on western medical training, the medical mindset and general hospital system.

On the flip side, it's useful to be aware of the huge social, psychological and emotional pressures against eating mainly raw foods. Food advertising, social norms, and the general lack of health awareness in our culture all contribute to the challenge and adventure of an eat more raw lifestyle. We know a heck of a lot about illness and disease simply because western medicine has studied illness and disease almost exclusively, at the expense of studying health. So, looking around us today, how much do we actually know about real, positive, vibrant health? How many ordinary people are truly healthy? And how much does our culture and medical system help us create real health? What is the 'normal' state of health? And why?

Looked at another way, health is a product of nature. So what natural laws determine our state of health? There must be some such natural laws - and knowing nature, they are probably simple.

Think for a moment about how much advertising there is for raw fruit and veg – think hard. That's right, virtually none! Meanwhile processed and junk food advertising is everywhere – often with marketing directly targeted at kids. Coca Cola and McDonalds are amongst the most well-known brand names in the world, deliberately pushed hard at the young, as the 'McLibel' court verdict showed[7]. Are they the ultimate symbols of the civilised, western good life? This says a lot about how much we value health in comparison with profit and a take-away lifestyle.

These foods are widely known to be unhealthy and are pushed, pushed, pushed at us, alongside the pressures of the heavy sell, addictive, high sugar, and high protein foods ... style-laden chocolate, ice-cream and coffee ads ... with bright packaging and give-away toys for the kids. All this bombards our minds and emotions, day in, day out. It's hard enough for any adults to resist, but then there's the parents of small children, and those small children themselves – *'we gotta catch 'em young if we're to increase our profits and protect brand value'*.

So much so that because of all the toys it includes with its children's meal packages McDonalds is classified as the world's largest 'toy distributor'[8]... No reason to wonder 'why?' To me this a blatant profit-oriented manipulation of children and parents emotions which is frightening to me given what we know about the long term effects of fast food on peoples' health – as was illustrated very graphically by the *Supersize Me* film. So how come such foods are allowed to be freely sold, whilst at the same time there are moves to restrict 'natural' medicines? A bizarre state of affairs indeed!

But let's remember that in many ways the legislators are as much the victims of this situation as anyone, and far from a picture of health themselves. Then there's vast vested commercial interests, the power of the food industry giants and pressure of industry lobbying to consider – which is very clearly described in the excellent book *The China Study*.[9] The truth is that it is

---

[7] Mr Justice Rodger Bell ruled that McDonald's endangered the health of their workers and customers by "misleading advertising", they "exploit children", they were "culpably responsible" in the infliction of unnecessary cruelty to animals, they were "antipathetic" to unionization and paid their workers low wages.

[8] "McDonalds distributes 1.5 billion toys annually around the world ... more than Toys R' Us! Obviously ... each happy meal comes with a toy. In the U.S. nine out of ten kids between the ages of 3 and 9 eat at McDonalds once a month" - source: http://www.omgfacts.com

[9] T Colin Campbell, *The China Study*, Benbella (2005).

patently unrealistic to expect our legislators or industry 'leaders' to sort out our health for us. We can argue they should, but it's 99.99% certain they won't! ... So who will do it for you?

There's a whole range of foods from the worst junk foods, through to various supposedly healthy snacks and sandwiches, many dosed with too much sugar and a range of 'killer' fats, that all work together to support the idea that processed cooked foods are perfectly 'normal'.[10] All of which means eating a whole lot of raw foods must be a bit 'weird' perhaps? Or perhaps not?

For some people, once they grasp the essence of a more 'natural', ecological or intuitive approach to food and health, it becomes easy to walk away from all this advertising of processed and industrialized 'garbage' food – and sometimes quite hurriedly!

As you come to sense more clearly the craziness of what goes on around food and health in our society, a vital and relatively easy first step is to walk away from the many processed foods that are so obviously unnatural and unhealthy. At the same time, think about the foods that you know are natural foods and healthy foods. From a fresh perspective it is clear that most of the very unhealthy foods are also more profitable foods; for the food producers, the illness and pharmaceutical drug industry, the supplement sellers and so on.

Meanwhile the most natural foods tend to sustain smaller businesses, local economies and appropriate farming systems, and are simply the most health creating foods. It *is* that simple.

Sickness and ill-health are sold to us as 'normal' and unavoidable - sometimes consciously, sometimes unconsciously. As a result we have innocently become a junk-and-processed-food-addicted society, largely unprotected from the consequences. With a massive and hugely expensive 'health' system, which has an infinite range of drugs for any condition, but which never heals, cures or solves the problem, instead hiding the symptoms whilst sustaining the sickness. If your health is taken from you then your freedom is reduced, and for some removed completely. Think about that. And the fear of illness greatly reduces our sense of freedom, making us feel we need constant easy access to doctors, hospitals and drugs, keeping us working away to keep up the medical insurance payments.

All this is a sales hype that can be very easy to walk away from when you have choices about where else you can head for. Once you understand that *you can actually take control of your own health*, then all this can change - and can be incredibly liberating.

So, eating a lot of raw foods can be a fad for some, but for the majority, an "eat more raw" lifestyle is the result of a genuine search for an improvement in their lifestyle – either for their own benefit or to benefit their relationship with the planet... and often both of course.

If you do choose to explore eating more raw foods then your lifestyle will change - changing you and the world around you. So in doing so, please understand that you are helping to create positive change, using your lifestyle to create numerous positive 'ripple effects'.

Kale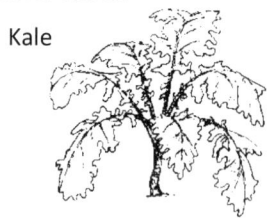

---

[10] Dr Udo Erasmus, *Fats that Heal Fats that Kill*, Alive Books (1993).

SUSTAINABILITY AND HEALTH – FAD OR FUTURE?

So what about sustainable living? Is that a passing fad, or our only option for the future? There's two key points to sustainability and health:

Firstly, *health and sustainability are essentially the same processes*, one applied to internal systems and the other applied to external systems – it is no coincidence that our culture is hugely successful at creating ill-health both in humans and in ecosystems, the environment and the planet as a whole. This system ill-health is a natural and inevitable outcome of our lack of understanding, our dominant patterns of thinking and our actions.

Secondly, *as a culture or civilization we have no choice but to create sustainability if we are to have a long term future* - although we may have to drop the 'S' word if we are to achieve it – achieving global whole health or 'real health' (ecological health, climate health, economic health, social health and individual health) is probably a better, more meaningful concept and state for us to pursue. If we are to reproduce successfully, the same goes for health.

In the meantime if you understand the essence of what creates health, then you can transfer that to understand the essence of what creates sustainability.

Sustainability (or whole health) is about living in ways that allow us to continue or maintain a certain quality of life, on a permanent basis. This in turn implies establishing a permanent (i.e. sustainable) agriculture and a sustainable culture (e.g. including an education system that teaches us how to live, work and play sustainably). In this sense, sustainable definitely means a naturally health creating agriculture and culture.

Sustainability, in its simplest definition, *is the ability-to-sustain*:

Sustain: *keep from falling or sinking, esp. for prolonged period; keep going continuously.*[11]

"... *ecologists have developed the concept of* resilience - *the ability of the system to maintain its structures and patterns of behaviour on the face of external disturbance i.e. its adaptability to change. This is usually distinguished from ecological* stability - *the ability of the system to maintain a relatively constant condition (its "equilibrium") ... in response to normal fluctuations and cycles in the surrounding environment. The basic properties for natural populations, communities and ecosystems are therefore* productivity *(in terms of numbers/biomass of individual species),* stability *(constancy) and* resilience *(sustainability)*"[12]

Similarly a state of health is a state of *dynamic equilibrium* (stability) which carries with it a high level of *resilience*, in terms of a *healthy immune system*. Ecosystems and habitats have immune systems too, so sustainable ways of living and working support and maintain the *ecological immune systems*, at both the local and planetary level – which is clearly in stark contrast to the ongoing weakening of ecological immune systems by western "civilised' industrial agriculture, resource exploitation and polluting forms of industrialisation in general.

---

[11] From the Concise Oxford English Dictionary.

[12] Pearce et al, *Blueprint for a Green Economy*, Earthscan, London (1995), p.40.

These are absolutely fundamental points to understand about *why* the current ways of thinking and doing simply cannot continue indefinitely, and are arriving at critical states of *chronic physical and ecological ill-health, at exactly the same time.*

So, with these definitions in mind, think for a moment about the parallels and similarities between 'sustainability' as a property of the wider environment, and 'health' (or healthiness) as a property of any organism, such as yourself. Read through the paragraph above in italics again, thinking about it as a description of the *healthiness* of an organism this time.

To give the definition above more meaning in relation to our individual and cultural lifestyles, their degree of sustainability can be defined as '*the extent to which that lifestyle can be supported by the planet's ecosystems and resources*'. So *sustainability means a lifestyle that can be entirely supported on an ongoing basis by the ecosystems and renewable resources of the planet, without causing significant unhealthy side effects elsewhere.*

And unsustainable means it can't be.

"*Sustainability means treating the planet as if we meant to stay*", Sir Crispin Tickell

This thinking has been well developed in the increasingly widely used and widely accepted technique of 'Ecological Footprinting', which indicates that the current western or UK lifestyle would need at least three planet Earths to sustain it, at current population levels, if we all shared the same lifestyle! The average American lifestyle would need around five planet Earths, with the bigger consumers greedily gobbling up the equivalent of eight or more planet Earths. So these levels of consumption are simply not sustainable, because we only have one planet.

Stabilizing climate change is one critical aspect of achieving sustainability, because we need dynamic stability. Most people do not yet fully understand or accept that climate change means *on-going and expanding dynamic instability* in weather patterns and extreme weather events, and therefore also in agriculture and food supply systems, *and* in diseases that thrive in the new climate, *and* in energy and travel infrastructure, *and* many, many other areas. It is increasingly clear that we have to reduce global carbon dioxide emissions by at least 80% to have a chance of stabilising climate change. Therefore, whether it's food growing and distribution, housebuilding or your own energy use at home and at work, if it isn't reduced by 80% then it isn't sustainable (unless you are already 80% below the average!). And based on current progress, or the lack of it, I suspect that by 2020, or 2025 at the latest, we'll be needing to cut emissions by 90%.

Moving from the unsustainable to the sustainable requires an understanding of the ripple effects of activities and relationships within these systems – climate systems, ecosystems, food growing systems, energy supply systems, as well as the internal ecology of our physiological systems. People talk about economic sustainability, social sustainability and environmental sustainability – or the sustainability of our food growing or energy supply systems. However, we can't achieve sustainability (or health) in any one of these systems without achieving it in the others - because the separation between the sub-systems is artificial, created by our minds.

So ideas of economic compensation for ecological damage work within an economic bubble, but are literally insane on a practical level. Such ideas arise from the fantastically disconnected conceptual modes of thinking that created all the problems in the first place, and which are constantly recreating, expanding and sustaining those problems. As an analogy, the rest of your body could be in good shape, but if your heart stops working the whole thing collapses – and there's no compensating the rest of your body if your heart breaks down ... or lungs, or liver.

The separation does not have reality in the world beyond our mind because these sub-systems are wholly interconnected, constantly affecting each other in ways we cannot comprehend if we try to separate them. What may seem an economically sustainable form of agro-industry quite simply is not if it's destroying the fertility of the soil, and the complexity of nature's interactions which cause pollination of crops, and sustain the vast complexity and productivity of insect and bacterial life. These things are interconnected 'holons', where coherent wholes (organisms) are also parts of larger coherent wholes (ecosystems), and wholes that are also made up of parts, which in themselves are also coherent wholes ... But this is all getting a bit theoretical, so it's time to sum up and move on:

In a nutshell: nature sustains life by creating and nurturing communities. No individual organism can exist in isolation ... Sustainability, therefore, is not an individual property but a property of an entire web of relationships ... This then is the profound lesson we need to learn from nature.[13]

Similarly we can say - *Health, therefore, is not an individual property but a property of an entire web of relationships.* This is the point of sustainability *and* health - we have to pursue them in numerous areas, and *we have to think and act sustainably and healthily in numerous areas, in a concerted and interconnected way if we are to have any hope of achieving healthy, sustainable outcomes.* This summarises the central message, method and inspiration of this book – so I suggest you re-read and reinforce it in your heart and mind.

The key is to understand that health and sustainability are essentially the same – one is primarily applied to an organism, ourselves, or our internal systems, whilst the other is applied to the external systems, the environment, economy and our culture as a whole.

An Alternative View of Sustainability ...

This we know; the Earth does not belong to humanity;
People belong to the Earth, this we know.
All things are connected.
Whatever befalls the Earth, befalls the people of the Earth.
We do not weave the web of life, we are merely part of it.
Whatever we do to the web, we do to ourselves.
The 'Chief Seattle Speech'[14]

To understand sustainability and how to create and live it, re-read the quote above again ... and again, and others of a similar nature. It is likely to be far more useful than technical definitions of sustainability for creating a deep understanding of what it means in practice.

---

[13] Fritjof Capra, *Landscapes of Learning*, in Resurgence, Sept/Oct 2004 – see also Fritjof Capra, *The Hidden Connections*, Flamingo (2005);

[14] Credited to Prof. Ted Perry, written for a radio play script, and based on a real speech by Chief Seattle.

In practice, one problem in shifting the western, developed nations to a more wise and sustainable path is that the vast majority of people no longer know how to grow food – whether individually or to serve local markets. They are trapped by that lack of knowledge, skills and confidence, therefore must take what they are given - lacking information, quality and true choice, as they feel unable to grow their own foods.

Permaculture (which is a system for designing sustainable lifestyles and sustainable living environments) is directly and deliberately designed to help us break out of this trap. It is also designed to enable us to enjoy more choice, more freedom and more fulfillment in life, whilst living responsibly. Permaculture is also about making carefully considered changes in our lives and living environments that are positive, constructive and sustainable. Its essence is to work with the patterns of nature and processes of life, health and sustainability rather than against them – working *with* nature, rather than against nature. And it is about designing and making changes in our lives, as a route to changing our world - taking responsibility for our lives, by creating naturally healthy and productive systems. And that is the essence of sustainability.

Permaculture is certainly highly adaptable. And judging by the enthusiastic way in which many people have taken up its ideas and applied them around the world if permaculture is a fad then it is a very useful and enjoyable one. So if you want to know more, then you'll learn much more from the permaculture section later in the book.

For now it is enough to know that sustainability and permaculture are concerned with producing healthy food in sustainable ways, how much and what types of energy we use, how much waste and pollution we produce and what we do with it, where we live, how we build or retrofit our homes and buildings, and the effects of our general lifestyle on people, the earth's ecosystems, species and atmosphere. Around 30% of all our sustainability impacts are estimated to be directly related to food; the ways we grow it, transport it, process it, pack it, cook it, dispose of it and so on. So food is a big piece of the sustainability jigsaw puzzle.

WHY RAW FOOD AND SUSTAINABILITY?

Why focus on eating more raw food and sustainability at the same time? Simple, because they go together so well. In fact, it's not about raw food or diet, it's about health and sustainability – which not only fit together well, at a fundamental level they are inseparable.

To explain further, one reason they go together is that they both work with nature. Working with nature to consciously create health and sustainability *involves working positively with the web of life*, inside your body and in the world around you.

This is about internal and external ecology, which are inextricably linked of course. In getting a feel for ecology why just look outside the body? If we *really* want to understand and practice ecology then we need to look at the ecology of the human body (and mind) as part of the ecology of the environment that the human body is a living, co-existing part of.

This book emerged because it's logical to set out these two contexts together – to link not separate them - as they are inseparable. It aims to encourage a thoroughly nourishing and fantastically fruitful exploration of natural, ecological approaches to health and sustainability! So most of this book is about the day to day practicalities of all this.

Personally, I eat mainly raw foods and have done so since autumn 1994. I've had many months and years when I've eaten only raw foods, usually mainly fruit, supplemented with dried fruit, nuts and seeds, and with one large salad a day, generally in the evening.

My intellectual reasons for eating as I do are guided by applying ecological reasoning and ethical considerations to my choices of what and how I eat. This is complemented by a healthy dose of research on diet, nutrition and lifestyle, looking at what naturally creates sickness, chronic illness and ill-health, as well as observation of what naturally creates health.

Equally importantly, alongside these intellectual reasons, are my intuitive reasons for eating as I do, guided by what *feels* more natural to me and what *feels* good to my body.

Meanwhile I've worked in the sustainability field since 1992, having studied it deeply both within my Masters degree (completed in '92) and through my own informal studies before then and after. I've investigated sustainability from many angles – buildings and construction, energy, food, ecology, health and so on - over many years, at many levels, from the personal and grassroots level, to local projects and policy, to regional projects and national strategy.

Linking health and sustainability is relevant to people everywhere, in all climates. A sustainable, *eat more raw* lifestyle may feel easier to achieve in warm climates where nature makes it easy to grow a wide variety of fruit and veg, and provides abundant solar energy. In sub-tropical, Mediterranean and tropical climates, forest gardens, community gardens, permaculture systems, organic market gardens and agroforestry can be easily designed to be both beautiful and bountiful; providing many types of vegetables, fruit and herbs all year round that are ideally suited to a high percentage raw diet. They can also provide building materials (timber, bamboo, etc.), fibres, soaps, oils and many other useful plant products.

In a temperate climate the variety is more limited, but still far greater than most people would imagine because the plant world is truly extraordinary and diverse. A sustainable temperate high raw food diet might consist fairly equally of salads, leafy greens and fruit, with a range of nuts, seeds and sprouted pulses, superfoods and 'food-state' supplements – a diet that can be very diverse, and much more enjoyable than one might think and certainly much healthier, more diverse and more sustainable than the typical western diet.[15]

If you want to see change in yourself and changes in the health and sustainability of the world outside you, it will help if you know what helps you understand how to do so. Do you need an image of vibrant health, true sustainability and how to get there? Do you need a sense of what true health and sustainability might feel like to your body and the feelings you need to help you get there? Or do you need a logical, factual understanding of what health and sustainability is and how to achieve it?[16] Explore this and you may find you can work it out for yourself.

---

[15] Vitamins and minerals need compatible organic substances to those they are surrounded by in their natural state for effective assimilation and ease of transportation throughout the body. 'Food State' nutrients are complexed in the appropriate materials, so that the body can recognise them as similar to a whole food (source: www.natures-own.co.uk).

[16] If you want to understand more about how your mind works I recommend *The Mind Map Book* by Tony Buzan, BBC Books (1995) and *From Frogs To Princes* by Bandler and Grinder, Eden Grove Editions (1990).

PART 2: THE PROBLEM – ILL HEALTH IS NATURAL

ACCEPTANCE OR RESPONSE–ABILITY?

Ill health is natural because ill-health is a natural outcome of any set of conditions and processes which are likely to create ill-health.

Agriculture, industry and the global-to-local economy play a massive role in shaping our environment, both the landscape we see and the cycles of carbon, oxygen and water which we do not see. Ultimately it is our ways of thinking and our values which shape that agriculture, those landscapes, the food industry, the local-to national-to-global food economy and those cycles of carbon, water and oxygen. In that sense it is our culture which is unsustainable, and which *'naturally' creates human and environmental ill-health* as symptoms of unsustainable thinking and unsustainable, unhealthy ways of living and working.

Conventional farming relies on highly manipulated plants which produce a high starch/sugar content. The plants are depleted in their mineral content because their resources are shifted to produce starch/sugar, and because the *available* minerals in the soil have been consistently depleted over the years - and demineralised food is a very important issue for our health. So, whilst *industrialised* agriculture produces huge *quantities* of 'food' it also does a great deal to deny us *genuine nutritional quality, balance and diversity.*

However, we *can* change all this. We can develop the ability and the motivation to respond positively.

PERSONAL AND PLANETARY HEALTH

Before we try to decide which path to health and sustainability we take it makes sense to recognise and accept where we are now in the 'personal and planetary health' landscape.

The WHO (World Health Organisation) definition of health is a *'state of complete mental, physical and social well being and not merely an absence of disease or infirmity'*. Based on this, and considering we take ourselves to be a scientifically and technologically advanced civilisation, what is the norm now for western people? Is it health, as defined by the WHO? What proportion of us achieve that WHO definition? Or even get close to it?

Virtually none do.

When health is something that benefits us all, individually and as a society, what does it say about our 'advanced' culture that it is so hugely *un*-successful at achieving the WHO definition of health? What does it say about our culture, and *its application of science*, that it is *so massively successful at creating chronic ill-health*?

If we are not healthy as a culture or as individuals, then what causes and effects deprive us of that 'complete state of well being'? And what can we do to fundamentally change that?

At the personal level, when it comes to food we are literally the 'consumers' of it, so it makes sense to think about what we are consuming – not just the food itself, but also the chain of effects that got it to your plate... the packaging, the processing, the deals with the suppliers, where it came from originally, the amount of energy, fossil fuels and pollution involved in getting it to you, the kind of landscape or wildlife habitat it creates (or destroys), the philosophy of the company that's selling and marketing it, and so on. And also the research that got it there.

Let's look at some known research on the effects of food on health. Firstly, please note that an extensive study by the American Medical Association *back in 1961* showed that vegetarians are dramatically healthier - clearly little was done to promote this scientifically determined conclusion. The excellent book by T Colin Campbell *The China Study* (2005) explains why, arising from his work as Emeritus Professor of Nutritional Biochemistry at Cornell University, and his many years involvement in and observation of US food and health committees.[17]

For those that need this kind of institutional scientific validation, numerous more recent studies are quoted on the Physicians Committee for responsible Medicine website:

"Harvard studies that included tens of thousands of women and men have shown that regular meat consumption increases colon cancer risk by roughly 300 percent.[8,9]

High-fat diets also encourage the body's production of estrogens, in particular, estradiol. Increased levels of this sex hormone have been linked to breast cancer. A recent report noted that the rate of breast cancer among premenopausal women who ate the most animal (but not vegetable) fat was one-third higher than that of women who ate the least animal fat.[10]

A separate study from Cambridge University also linked diets high in saturated fat to breast cancer.[11]

One study linked dairy products to an increased risk of ovarian cancer. The process of breaking down the lactose (milk sugar) into galactose evidently damages the ovaries.[12]

Daily meat consumption triples the risk of prostate enlargement. Regular milk consumption doubles the risk and failure to consume vegetables regularly nearly quadruples the risk.[13]

Vegetarians avoid the animal fat linked to cancer and get abundant fiber, vitamins, and phytochemicals that help to prevent cancer. In addition, blood analysis of vegetarians reveals a higher level of "natural killer cells," specialized white blood cells that attack cancer cells.[14"]

And, for those that want them, the references for the above are:

8. Giovannucci E, Rimm EB, Stampfer MJ, Colditz GA, Ascherio A, Willett WC. Intake of fat, meat, and fiber in relation to risk of colon cancer in men. *Cancer Res.* 1994;54:2390-2397.

9. Willett WC, Stampfer MJ, Colditz GA, Rosner BA, Speizer FE. Relation of meat, fat, and fiber intake to the risk of colon cancer in a prospective study among women. *N Engl J Med.* 1990;323:1664-1672.

10. Cho E, Speigelman D, Hunter DJ, Chen WY, Stampfer MJ, Colditz GA, Willett WC. Premenopausal fat intake and risk of breast cancer. *J Natl Cancer Inst.* 2003;95:1079-1085.

11. Bingham SA, Luben R, Welch A, Wareham N, Khaw KT, Day N. Are imprecise methods obscuring a relation between fat and breast cancer? *Lancet.* 2003;362:212-214.

---

[17] T Colin Campbell, *The China Study*, Benbella (2005).

12. Cramer DW, Harlow BL, Willett WC. Galactose consumption and metabolism in relation to the risk of ovarian cancer. *Lancet.* 1989;2:66-71.
13. Araki H, Watanabe H, Mishina T, Nakao M. High-risk group for benign prostatic hypertrophy. *Prostate.* 1983;4:253-264.
14. Malter M, Schriever G, Eilber U. Natural killer cells, vitamins, and other blood components of vegetarian and omnivorous men. *Nutr Cancer.* 1989;12:271-278.

That kind of science can be quoted endlessly - it's been there for years. Yet the US, UK and most western populations *have terrible levels of chronic ill-health*. Yes, the research *should* be making a difference, but the reality is that it is not. Arguably this is because of a combination of political and corporate vested interests, alongside a culture of ignorance, laziness and personal irresponsibility for health. So, if we want to take responsibility for our own health in this situation there is actually a great deal that *we can do*, and a great deal of research we can learn from.

There is a huge amount of evidence and experience that shows the numerous benefits of eating a high-percentage-raw diet. Leslie and Susannah Kenton's excellent book *The New Raw Energy* details many *historical* research studies, including:[18]

- The work of the Swiss Physician Max Bircher–Brenner in studying the great healing benefits of 'living foods' as he called them.
- The German physician Max Gerson's work, initially on migraine, then on the 'incurable' disease lupus, and most famously on cancer as detailed in his book *A Cancer Therapy: Results of Fifty Cases.*[19]
- The Danish physician Kristine Nolfi's successful personal battle against breast cancer.
- The rigorous work of the scientist Arnold Ehret on fasting and 'the mucousless diet'.
- The work of US dentist Weston A Price on nutrition and physical degeneration.
- And the American juice therapy and colon irrigation expert Dr Norman Walker who was physically and mentally healthy and active up to the day of his death, when he died peacefully in his sleep at home, some say at the age of 99, some at 106!

So what about more up to date research?

The significant distortion of a) research funding and b) the application of science by the food, medical and drug industries means that *modern institutional scientific research on* health creation *is few and far between* – if you don't understand that yet, then this may not be the book for you. However, a course such as the Masters programme in *Professional Coaching, Mentoring and Consultancy for Health and Wellbeing* at Bath Spa Univeristy could be for you, as it includes modules such as *'The Principles & Evidence Base for Health and Wellbeing'*. Also T Colin Campbell's *The China Study* could be the book for you.

---

[18] Leslie & Susannah Kenton, The New Raw Energy, Vermillion (1995).

[19] Max Gerson, *A Cancer Therapy: Results of Fifty Cases*, Gerson Institute (1958).

INSTITUTIONAL SCIENCE V'S THE BLATANTLY FLIPPING OBVIOUS

To finish this section, let's ask, *where is it we find shining examples of health and well-being?* Is it in the institutional health research community? Or is it within the natural health movement? Between those two communities, *which has undertaken the most valid and valuable research in generating a* real *understanding of health creation?* Please take a moment and consider these fundamentally important questions.

Within the natural health and raw foods movement there are numerous experts, whose expertise is based on *years and years of experience, self-experimentation and observation.* These include in the USA Dr Gabriel Cousens, Dr Douglas Graham, Dr Joel Robbins and Dr Brian Clements, as well as more outspoken and charismatic characters such as David Wolfe. Meanwhile, the UK movement has its own identity with Sharon Holdstock, better known as 'Shazzie', Karen Knowler, Kate Wood, Mike Nash, Funky Raw Magazine and the Festival of Life. A fairly strong movement in Germany, with a more mature character, has roots that go back to the natural health movement of the nineteenth century.

The pioneers and advocates in these movements *have studied and researched in great detail the nutrition and lifestyles that naturally create and support health, and have drawn clear and consistent conclusions.* That is their primary personal interest, and it is what drives many of them as passionate educators in the field of natural health and nutrition. They have all understood that *a) the health creation systems of the human body and b) the immune system function much more effectively when they are fed by a diet that is essentially natural.*

They know from *direct personal experience over many years* that raw plant foods are excellent sources of all the nutrients they need for vibrant health. This isn't theory – this is conclusions drawn from experience of the pleasures and advantages of vibrant health. To emphasise this point, David Wolfe wisely points out that if you want to be successful in creating excellent health you simply have to seek out, study and copy those that are supremely healthy.

Whilst the natural health and raw food movements have a lot to offer, do shop around in terms of who you listen to or use as a source of advice and guidance. And look for those that have more to their life and their message than just food! Also be aware that many spiritual traditions also recognise the benefits of simple natural foods and/or fasting. So this knowledge is not new; it's been around for thousands of years, although it's been a little hidden until recently. It is tried, tested and proven, with its effects observed and repeated again and again ... even if conventional science has not studied it much (which means scientists have not been funded / financed by companies or government to study health creation – *instead* they *are* used, and paid more, to apply science to the industrialised production of highly processed foods).

So it is worth considering research into a) the successes of conventional medicine, and b) the life expectancy of humans around the world. Dr Joel Wallach recorded a fascinating and famous talk entitled *Dead Doctors Don't Lie* in 1994 (and book)[20], and was a specialist vet before he went on to train as a doctor. His conclusions from this research were that nutritional deficiency

---

[20] For information on the tape of the talk and the book see www.wallachonline.com/dead_doctors.htm – said to be the most popular health lecture in history, with around 46 million copies of the tape sold worldwide.

– particularly mineral deficiency - is a critical cause of illness and death, through the conditions that consistently arise from nutritional deficiencies.

Dr Wallach emphasises that the scientifically accepted view is that the genetic potential for longevity of human beings suggests we should live to around 120 to 140 years old and then die of natural causes. Clearly, not the norm. Dr Wallach has campaigned for many years against what he calls the fraud of the medical industry. He suggests there is great value in treating yourself, rather than putting your health in the hands of medical doctors who are simply *not trained to believe that medical conditions can be cured*, but who are trained *to prescribe expensive drugs to alleviate (or hide) the symptoms* of those medical conditions.

Dr Wallach has practiced for many years using nutrition with his patients, stating that if they followed his advice properly they were certain to add many healthy years to their life, and 'save a gob of money' in the process. In his 1994 lecture he quotes a 3 year study by consumer activist Ralph Nader (published in 1993) on the causes of death in US hospitals. This study states that '300,000 Americans are killed each year in hospitals alone as a result of medical negligence'. Nader compared this shocking annual statistic to the 10 years of the Vietnam War, where US military losses were around 56,000, leading to vast protests and demonstrations. Yet, Nader's study states that around *five times* that many people were 'being killed' *each year* in America's own hospitals by medical error or negligence. And when this is compared as an annual rate of death, this means about 50 times as many people were dying each year from 'iatrogenic' causes (i.e. effects of medical error) compared with the number of Vietnam deaths each year. With no mass protest about the hospital deaths. Why?

And in the early 21st century, heart disease is the number one cause of death in the US, and cancer the number two cause, with the number three cause, killing nearly a quarter of a million people a year, being misdiagnosis and prescribed medicine as the following shows:

The JOURNAL of the AMERICAN MEDICAL ASSOCIATION (JAMA) Vol 284, No 4, July 26th 2000 article written by Dr Barbara Starfield, MD, MPH, of the Johns Hopkins School of Hygiene and Public Health, shows that medical errors may be the third leading cause of death in the United States.

The report apparently shows there are 2,000 deaths/year from unnecessary surgery; 7000 deaths/year from medication errors in hospitals; 20,000 deaths/year from other errors in hospitals; 80,000 deaths/year from infections in hospitals; 106,000 deaths/year from non-error, adverse effects of medications - these total up to 225,000 deaths per year in the US from iatrogenic causes which ranks these deaths as the # 3 killer.

Iatrogenic is a term used when a patient dies as a direct result of treatments by a physician, whether it is from misdiagnosis of the ailment or from adverse drug reactions used to treat the illness. (drug reactions are the most common cause).

Source: unedited extract from the Cancer Cure Foundation website [21]

---

[21] Source: http://www.cancure.org/medical_errors.htm

An article titled *Death by Medicine* by three medical doctors and two PhDs on the Center for Sustainable Medicine website (http://www.sustainablemedicine.org/) suggest the figures could be much higher, with an annual cost of unnecessary or harmful medical intervention estimated at $282 billion.

In the UK the reporting of such information is grossly inadequate, so the gathering of information on the harm and cost of medical treatments is virtually impossible. However, we can briefly look at what we do know about the norms of UK 'health' and illness statistics:

How things are...
In England in 2010:
- over a quarter of adults (26% of both men and women aged 16 or over) were classified as obese (Body Mass Index 30kg/m2 or over);
- 31% of boys and 29% of girls (aged 2 to 15) were classed as either overweight or obese
- around one in ten pupils aged 4-5 years were classified as obese (9.4%)
  source: http://www.hscic.gov.uk
- In 2013, bowel cancer was the second most common cause of cancer death in the UK and over 15,700[2] people die each year; that's someone every 30 minutes
  source www.bowelcanceruk.org.uk
- The Human Fertilisation and Embryology Authority (HFEA) estimates that around one in seven couples in the UK experience difficulty conceiving (ONS, 2009) - the delicacy and sophistication of our reproductive system means it is inevitably something that suffers in conditions which naturally create ill-health.

Rankings of years of life lost by illness (1 year is best, 19 year is worst)						
Country	Heart disease	Stroke	Lung cancer	Breast cancer	COPD	Cirrhosis
UK	14	13	12	18	17	11
USA	18	5	16	8	19	15

Note: COPD represents lung diseases, including chronic bronchitis and emphysema. Years of life lost is the number of years early a person dies compared to life expectancy.

So there's something significant going on here! This all emphasizes that whilst hospitals and the medical system are vital for treating severe accidents or life-threatening situations, *they do not create healthy people.* In their current form they never will. They are not and never will be places to go *if you want to create health. You have to go somewhere else.* This is really important to recognize and accept if you are genuinely interested in creating real health.

It is also worth noting that whilst higher incomes generally lead to longer life expectancy, it is also the case that wealth does not equal health. Hugely wealthy people die of heart disease and cancer in their 50s and 60s like the rest. Sir James Goldsmith, a billionaire financier, who was one of Britain's wealthiest men, died aged 64 of a heart attack, said to have been brought on by pancreatic cancer. Wealth can pay to keep you alive in an unhealthy state because you can afford the very best treatment in that bad state of health. But wealth does not make you healthy. Whilst health care insurance and treatment for ill-health may be expensive, health itself is not. Health can be achieved on a very low income, a middle income or a high income.

True, natural health does not discriminate, as can be seen from studies of the often very poor tribes that live long and very healthy lives. Economically poor cultures around the world are generally far healthier than us westerners - although they normally face much greater challenges from contagious diseases related to their living conditions and environment (such as malaria and water borne diseases), rather than diet. This brings their life expectancy down. Lack of food and poverty-induced malnutrition are still major, major problems in many areas around the world, often where debt to the west has forced changes in agricultural systems away from local self-reliance, towards cash-crops ... but that's another story.

So what is the point to these facts and statistics? The point is to question, what is really happening with our health? And with your health? The point is to ask: *in terms of what we can control in our life, what makes the difference between health and longevity, poor health, chronic illness and an early death? Can I reasonably expect an outcome different to the norm, if I do what others normally do?*

The point is to ask: is it a simple or complex difference? Is institutional science most likely to help me, or can I help myself? And, the point is also to ask yourself: does this matter to me, or my family? And if it does, *what can I, personally, do about it?*

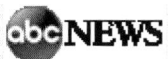
KAIJING XIAO, Friday, September 19, 2014, BEIJING --

China has fined the British pharmaceuticals giant GlaxoSmithKline (GSK) $488.8 million (3 billion Yuan) for a "massive bribery network" to get doctors and hospitals to use its products ... The fine was the biggest ever imposed by a Chinese court.

The court gave Mark Reilly, former head of GSK Chinese operations, a three-year prison sentence with a four-year reprieve, which meant he is set to be deported instead of serving his time in a Chinese jail. His co-defendants received two to four years prison sentences with reprieves.

Source: http://abcnews.go.com/International/glaxosmithkline-gsk-fined-4888-million-massive-bribery-network/story?id=25624684

The above merely indicates the outcomes that our dominant economic and corporate structures tend to create, whether they come to the surface or not, whether in banking or pharmaceuticals. The question is, when it comes to *your* health, where do you want to place your trust?

THE TRUE COSTS OF INDUSTRIAL FOOD PRODUCTION SYSTEMS

- 1 000 tonnes of water are consumed to produce one tonne of grain
- 10 energy units are spent for every 1 energy unit of food on our dinner table
- 1 000 energy units are used for every 1 energy unit of processed food
- 17% of the total US energy use goes into food production & distribution, accounting for more than 20% of all US transport; this excludes energy used in import & export
- 20% of all greenhouse gases in the world come from current agriculture
- US$318 bn taxpayer's money subsidized agriculture in advanced OECD countries in 2002 - while more than 2 billion subsistence farmers tried to survive on $2/day
- 90% of the agricultural subsidies benefit corporations and big farmers growing food for export; while 500 family farms close down every week in the United States
- Subsidized surplus food dumped on developing countries creates poverty, hunger and homelessness on a massive scale
Source: Sustainable World Initiative, http://swinitiative.com/
Now that's what I call unsustainable.

SOME BENEFITS OF SUSTAINABLE FOOD PRODUCTION SYSTEMS

- 2- to 10-fold energy saving on switching to low-input/organic agriculture
- 5-15% fossil-fuel emissions offset by carbon sequestering organically managed soil
- 50 to 92% reduction in carbon dioxide emission from the soil on switching from conventional tillage to no-till agriculture
- 5 tonnes of CO_2 emission disappear with every tonne of nitrogen fertilizer phased out
- 2-3-fold crop yield increase using compost in Ethiopia, exceeding chemical fertilizers
- US organic farming performs as well or better than conventional industrial farming
- Small farms are 2 to 10 times more productive than larger farms
- Organic farms support significantly more birds, bats, invertebrates and wild plants than conventional farms in Europe
- Organic foods contain more vitamins, minerals and other micronutrients than conventionally produced foods
- 1 000 or more community-supported farms across US and Canada bring $36m income per year directly to the farms
- £50-78m go directly into the pocket of farmers trading in some 200 established local farmers' markets in the UK
- Buying food in local farmers' market generates twice as much for the local economy than buying food in supermarket chains
- Money spent with a local supplier is worth 4 times that spent with non-local supplier
Source: Sustainable World Initiative - www.indsp.org/SustainableWorldInitiative.php

DIETARY CARBON AND CLIMATE CHANGE IMPACTS (CO2 + METHANE)

The FAO estimates that 18% of global emissions result from livestock, while food system emissions are estimated to be around 24% of all human emissions – with 12% from agricultural production, 9% from farming induced deforestation, and 3% from refrigeration, freight, etc.

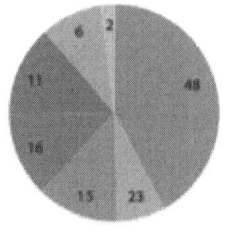

- Agriculture – 48%
- Transport & packaging – 23%
- Primary & secondary processing -15%
- Retail & catering - 16%
- Domestic food management – 11%
- Waste disposal – 6%
- Fertilizer manufacture – 2%

Source: Climate Change and Food Systems, Vermeulen, Campbell and Ingram, 2012.

Impacts vary greatly depending on the type of food economy in any country, with carbon impacts being very much higher for large scale, fertilizer fed, machinery harvested, long distance transported, highly processed foods i.e. most of a conventional western diet. Estimates of the carbon impacts are diet are inevitably generalized, however, what is clear is that meat in particular, and also dairy produce have significantly higher carbon impacts. So, as indicated below a US-style vegan diet has less than half the impacts of a US-meat lover.

Comparison of Carbon FOODprints (tonnes CO2 emissions)

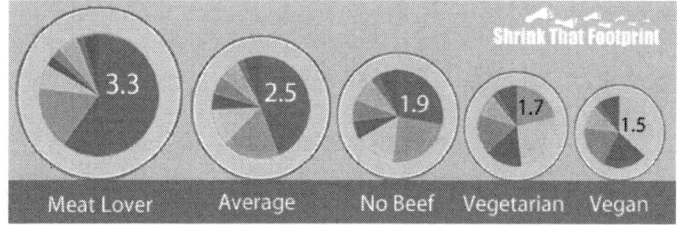

Source: http://shrinkthatfootprint.com/food-carbon-footprint-diet

Basically, the more local seasonal and organic produce (without transport and industrial fertilizer's carbon impacts) and the more homegrown produce, the better. We also know
- Legumes have very low impacts, even if imported, so sprouting has a very low impact;
- Seasonal temperate fruits have a very low impact, as do locally produced veg;
- Even imported bananas and oranges have a relatively low impact.

Mike Berners-Lee's book *How Bad Are Bananas?* is great for understanding your dietary and other impacts – and showing bananas aren't bad! From that and other sources, it is clear that *an eat more raw diet, with a good slice of home-grown and locally sourced produce will definitely be under the 1.5-1.7tonnes CO2 emissions, nearer to 1tCO2e, with clear potential to be much less the more you grow for yourself and the more you choose carefully. To me it is not a question of measuring your diet impacts in detail (although for some that will be fascinating), it is question of getting a good sense of what has low impacts, and choosing accordingly.*

HEALTH AND SUSTAINABILITY - WHERE ARE WE HEADING?

We are getting close to the positive, action-oriented part of this book, which is most of it. So hold on for a few more pages whilst we complete the story of health in pretty much any western nation, painting as accurate a picture as possible of where we are now and where we are heading, so that we can accurately determine where we might prefer to be and how to get there.

If we want to know where we are heading in terms of sustainability and health trends, when we pull together the current trends around us we see:

- Less traditional diseases, but very high rates of *chronic ill-health* (misleadingly called 'lifestyle disease'), and serious rising obesity levels including at a younger age.
- More people surviving longer in a fundamentally unhealthy state, with many years of chronic ill-health *expected* for most people - with *widespread acceptance of unhealthiness and chronic illness* as being normal, with a right to ongoing treatment – and the massive cost of this bringing great profit to a few.
- Rising global economic centralization in major corporations, major economic uncertainty and instability, an ongoing shift towards the over-riding global influence of the 'financial industries', with dubious new financial 'products' continually emerging and growing like viruses, alongside tax havens, secrecy laws and *massive* tax avoidance.[22]
- High levels of crime and high levels of fear of crime.
- The illegal drugs trade is one of the biggest industries around the world, *especially in the most developed, 'civilised' societies (*benefiting from secrecy laws & tax havens).
- The legal drugs and pharmaceutical trade *also* one of the biggest world industries.
- The breakdown of communities and a growing 'fortress culture'.
- Widespread disillusionment and lack of confidence in 'the system', politics and media.
- A lack of confidence in our health (physical, environmental, political and economic) ... and therefore a lack of confidence in our future.
- Environmental degradation, global desertification and gradual climate change.

This seems like one-way traffic, and if the trends continue it has only one possible outcome – more and more and more of the same, because if you look at each of these trends there really is nothing much to suggest any realistic possibility of turning any one of these trends around.

If we look at how we produce our food, half the world's river water is being used to irrigate crops – which has massive impacts on the natural ecosystems dependent on those rivers. Potatoes are most efficient large-scale crop in agro-industrial water-use terms – they need 500 litres of water per kg of potatoes, whilst chickens need 3,500 litres/kg, and beef requires 100,000 litres/kg (i.e. 100 tonnes of water for just 1kg of beef). In East Anglia (UK) for every 1 ton of wheat harvested, about 5 tons of soil is lost. At least 80% of arable land in Britain is used to grow fodder for animals.

---

[22] See the excellent book *Treasure Islands*, by Nicholas Shaxton for more info.

It's not all bad though! The future we create depends on how we collect and use the information and knowledge at our disposal. Things are changing, because *they have to change*. We have never had more information available. Wisdom, however, depends on how we *select* and *use* that information. Books like *The Tipping Point* (Malcolm Gladwell, 2000) and *The Hidden Connections* (Fritjof Capra, 2002) can help us understand how change can happen successfully and sometimes rapidly. U-Theory and other tools are also helping people to understand that it is now essential, and much more helpful to us, that we *learn from the emerging future*, more than just learning from the past, as we have done. So *we have to learn from the emerging future of natural health and sustainability*. We need to *create and expand the possibility of health creation and sustainability*, for ourselves and for others.

Our society is over-loaded with information, whilst at the same time having a distinct lack of wisdom. In the sea of information, we drown in quantity and 'information garbage', with quality becoming more and more diluted. But we can learn to swim through it.

To *create* health as individuals or as a culture we (obviously) have to *learn how to create health first*. *Learning implies changes* in how we do things – it is not just accumulation of facts. The outcomes of learning depend on our thinking and values motivating us to change. Learning also implies that we accept we have something to learn – intellectual humbleness as opposed to intellectual arrogance or naivety. When it comes to sustainability and health, nature is our best and only teacher – so we need to learn from nature.

Creating health is not rocket science – it is do-able. It is a question of learning about nature, but not in a reductionist way. Western societies are dominated by technology – when we do learn from nature there is usually another human being, a computer or a book in between us and nature. We don't realise that the vehicle that we are travelling in provides the best lessons. *You are nature, embodied in human form.* Through our continual interaction with life, the universe and everything, we are all plugged into nature and evolution.

We are the universe looking at itself; consciousness embodied in the human body is the universe and nature attempting to understand itself and consciously interact with itself. Are we yet conscious of and making the most of that fact? Where do you see us heading? Do you want to join others and change direction to a path with hope of taking us towards a healthy, sustainable and fulfilling culture? A starting point is to feed better quality information into yourself, and the systems you are part of.

LIFE IN THE 21st CENTURY

As a society where are we heading and where do we want to be?

We know western life expectancy is typically between 50 and 80 years (e.g. US and UK average about 75 years) – typically with the last 10 to 12 years including suffering one or more serious degenerative diseases. Meanwhile it's scientifically accepted that the human body is capable of living healthily to around 120 to 130 years.

This means that the typical western lifestyle denies most of us - including you and me - virtually half of our life! If you follow the normal path something is killing you, giving you chronic illness, 40, 50 or 60 years before you are meant to die. Linked to declining nutritional quality, this is said to be the first generation where many parents will see their children die before them. This is where we are heading unless we change course – which we can quite easily do.

A POSITIVE VISION

We can gain excellent nutrition and health if we really start to think carefully, and start to *consciously design and create our food growing systems, diets and lifestyles to give us nutrition and lifestyles that naturally and automatically create health.*

And if you or anyone you are close to thinks this is unrealistic, then sit down and take a really long hard look at the current trends in *chronic ill health and healthcare costs* detailed in the last few pages. Think about the vision of where these trends will take us. How realistic is it to think we can sustain those trends *and growing costs* for another 5, 10 or 20 years?

Imagine how things will change if at least 50% of what we eat is whole organic fruit (depending on where you live this might include many varieties and flavours of apples, avocados, apricots, pears, oranges, mangos, grapes, melons, gojis and other berries) and vibrant, organic, mineral rich veg and salads, freshly picked from the garden or local farm or market garden every day. Surely this is at least part of a vision for health that we can all agree to? How would this change water demand, chemical use, soil fertility and soil loss? How would it affect our health?

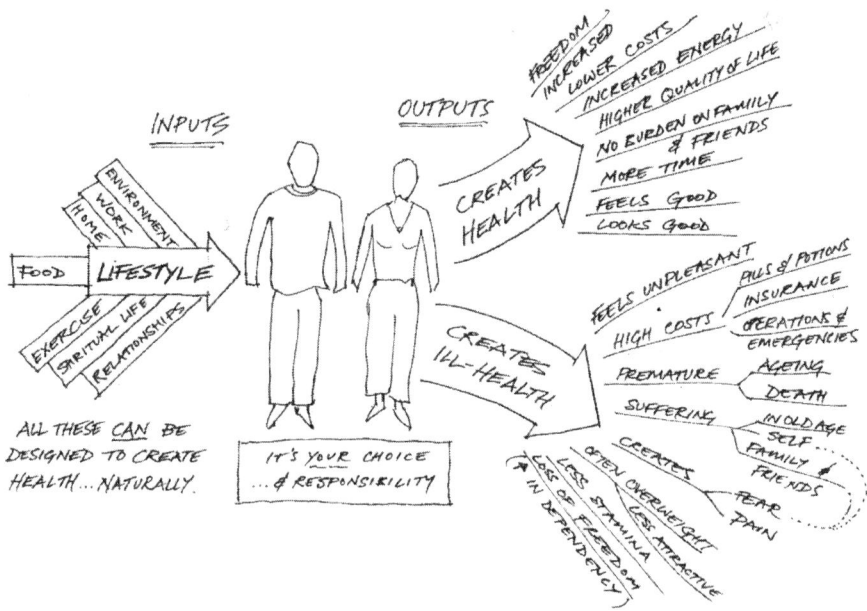

How would it affect your life and your health if you made these changes in your life? How might those changes then positively affect others around you?

Health and sustainability are totally dependent on our ability and willingness to a) learn and b) take action. Our current path is very clearly *not* achieving health or sustainability, so we have to learn a lot, and take action. The information is here with us now, we simply have to *use it* and *act on it* more wisely (and not just study it!). Something has to shift if we are to break the unhealthy and fundamentally unsustainable continuum. To change the strange loop, we have to step in and make decisions; make a firm choice and take action to create change. A key element of this is to develop a positive vision of a naturally healthy and sustainable life for yourself, within your vision a naturally healthy and sustainable culture.

So let's use our understanding of the deeper nature of the problem to create and implement sustainable and healthy solutions – positive, conscious, creative responses to our current situation.

CREATING REAL HEALTH

Our picture of health and sustainability can change, *when we do the painting of it for ourselves*. If we are to develop any kind of wholeness in health we will need a personalized package that creates health in mind, body, spirit and emotions. This may need you to rewrite your traditional stories about yourself and your society, and to *change your goals*. This might include:

1. Thou shalt consume at least 50% raw, life-giving, health creating foods, with intelligent use of knowledge of their benefits and effects.
2. Thou shalt regularly use meditation, massage and stress relief or relaxation techniques.
3. Thou shalt enjoy exercise and good breathing – yoga, tai chi, the Five Tibetans, etc.
4. Thou shalt enjoy clean, fresh air and water.
5. Thou shalt use and participate in action-learning groups, support groups such as co-counselling and groups focused on positive life changes.
6. Thou shalt engage in community for shared child care, friendship and diversity – a move to diverse, natural health-creating communities and sustainable extended families.
7. Thou shalt use a range of physical and emotional complimentary therapies, if needed.
8. Thou shalt enjoy artistic and creative activities.
9. Thou shalt enjoy and sustain a spiritual openness to growth and exploration.
10. Thou shalt enjoy plenty of opportunities for contact with nature, plants and the soil.

Oh, and laughter of course! We need to be serious about including that!

With such a package of mutually beneficial health creating activities, a revolution in personal and planetary health will gradually and naturally result, and the illness and dependency of conventional consumer society will evolve to something more positive, more healthy and more sustainable. All you have to do is sense how to set the creative, healthy forces of nature free in your life as a whole, and in its various elements that make up the whole. And then take practical, achievable steps to make it happen.

Here we go...

PART 3: THE SOLUTION – HEALTH IS NATURAL

INTERCONNECTEDNESS

If you sit in a quiet sunny spot in the garden, or look out at a park or distant hillside, or even just take a really good look at your window box, if you ponder about western science and the spiritual philosophies of both east and west you will find a whole lot of differing views of creation that generally all tell us that everything is connected.

This almost universal scientific and spiritual view of life tells us that creation is not something separate, it is here and now, and it is the world we live in day-by-day by-day... it is us, and we are it... nature, evolution. And both science and many spiritual traditions tell us that 'reality' often differs from our perception of it – often quite significantly.

We are told from an early age in school about atoms and molecules and so on. We are told that we and everything else, even the clear air around us, is all made up of this 'stuff-that-is-not-stuff', these atoms and molecules. And what's more about 99.9% of those molecules and fundamental particles are simply energy and nothingness.

So at what point does the oxygen in the air we breathe become part of us? When do the plants we eat stop being part of the environment and become our food? And at what point does the food we eat become part of us? We respond to our environment and our environment responds to us. We shape each other. Where is the division then, if one is part of the other and the 'other' part of one? Is 'nature' outside or in? Or is it both?

In this sense it is scientifically and spiritually accurate to state that you and your environment are what you eat – the one both creates and is created from the other. However, we are certainly not *only* what we eat!

WORKING WITH NATURE: A PRACTICAL PHILOSOPHY FOR SUSTAINABLE AND HEALTHY LIVING

'Working with nature, not against it' is a basic principle of ecology and sustainability[23].

The principle of working with nature provides a practical foundation for a healthy and sustainable philosophy for life. Personally, I have felt deep concern about the state of the world and mankind for many years, whilst at the same time constantly seeing the awesome creative potential of humanity. Much of that potential appears to be squashed or misdirected, so I really believe that we can and should create steady improvements for ourselves, our children and grandchildren. The idea of economic growth aims for this, however in its current form it is just not a sustainable and evolutionary path for humanity – unless our economic systems change radically ... which is possible.

---

[23] Distilled into this simple phrase by Bill Mollison, the founder of permaculture.

If we really want a positive sustainable path, either we need to adjust some of our economic priorities, or we have to change our lifestyles and our individual and social priorities – or do both of course. And we can certainly do this at an individual level, which then influences the social level.

To me evolution (whether biological or socio-cultural) means a significant positive development in our nature. Given the situation we are in at present, for humanity this includes consciously using the vast amounts of information, knowledge and experience we have, much more wisely, efficiently and effectively.[24] It means becoming more aware of the unique nature of our bodies as living systems, our consciousness, our patterns of understanding - and our significant patterns of mis-understanding – as well as our patterns of choices and the effects of those choices (including the choices we tend to run away from or resist).

Working with nature in a sophisticated way, means understanding nature and evolution to such an extent that it becomes obvious that the most positive path is to *work with nature inside and out*. To do this we need to create a positive vision of where we want to be in the future, as well as a clear sense of the practical steps we need to take to start us on that path.

As a first step we need to understand how to live in a changing and challenging world, in order to become much more confident and positive about dealing with this. This is where personal development, practical solutions like permaculture and confidence about our health are so valuable. What do you see when you take a look at the future we are heading towards? Would you like to feel safer and more secure about your future and the future of the world as a whole? You can if you make choices that take you in that direction.

A philosophy of working with nature is all about the realities of how we go forward towards health and sustainability now. It's about working with the creative, productive energy of life and nature to meet our own needs, by understanding the needs of our children, the next generation, and the next seven generations (to borrow a Native American way of thinking). 'Working with nature' is rooted in the practical realisation that the way we think and act now creates our future. Its deepest roots are in a sense of nature and of biological and social evolution that is beyond words. As a philosophy and way of life it seeks diversity, abundance, beauty and natural organic growth – a balance of intellect and intuition. It works with the natural flows, patterns and energies that naturally create these desirable outcomes. Working with nature means, for example, a recognition that creating beauty in what we do is really, really good for us in a practical sense, and is therefore very important e.g. beautiful food, homes, neighbourhoods and towns or cities.

Working with nature does not mean using 'human nature' as an excuse for our destructive and not so desirable behaviour – or as an excuse for having mediocre aspirations. It means recognising and building on the creative and inspirational nature of our behaviour. Nature always has the capacity to learn, adapt, grow and change. And for most of our 'civilised' history humanity has accepted that civilising ourselves includes an evolution of our values and activities, and the thinking and typical behaviour of our culture, as we learn, grow and change. So why should that

---

[24] i.e. an evolution of 'Information Technology' into 'Wisdom Technology', meaning the wise processing of the vast amounts of variable quality information our culture churns out, much of it unhelpful or a distraction, rather than significantly and easily useful – if you want to develop wisdom technology, please do!

stop? Legal and religious systems, and spiritual philosophies, developed to uphold the values that were seen as being 'right' and proper at the time. But evolution doesn't stop, so I feel that our thinking, values and actions should still be evolving, and I see nature as an important guide for this type of conscious evolution.

Where do you see our values going in the present age of civilisation? Do you feel we are making progress in creating a more caring world?

Personally, I feel that respecting all forms of life is important; human, animal and plant life. These values don't make me 'better' than someone that does kill, but I do feel 'better' in myself as a vegetarian (although not in a smug way).[25] I have found it feels better to me, in my relationship with the web of life and creation. I've also found that being vegetarian or vegan is a surprisingly easy and enjoyable on a path towards a compassionate life.

Inevitably such issues are personal choices which depend on the particular information, guidance and experiences we chance upon or seek out along our life's path. I know that I now feel better informed in my choices – my inner feelings and confidence about those choices are also much stronger.

BRIEF INTERLUDE: IF IT'S GOOD ENOUGH FOR GANDHI

A lot of people are interested in celebrities who are 'into' particular lifestyles or fashions. There's a particularly well known person that comes to mind when thinking of the 'eat more raw' lifestyle, although I wouldn't call this person a celebrity ... although he has been viewed by many as one of the most admirable and inspirational people who lived in the 20th century (born in the 19th).

How many people know that Mohandas K Gandhi, better known as Mahatma Gandhi or simply Gandhi, was a long term raw fooder, eating a simple essentially fruitarian diet for much of his life?

Gandhi was greatly influenced by the natural hygienists in the 1920's, and as a result he saw his exploration of diet and health as one his key 'experiments with the truth' - these experiments formed a foundation stone of his approach to life. Indeed this story is told in **M K Gandhi: An Autobiography, The Story of My Experiments with Truth,** *an excellent read which details much of his experiments with diet and fasting.*

Gandhi saw raw nutrition as essential in pursuing a path to both physical and spiritual health, strength and purification, although he did not see it as a sufficient path on its own. Gandhi's four fundamental values were:

- *a pursuit of truth (including and impossible without aiming for complete truth to and with oneself);*
- *the simplification of life and his needs to a essential (basic) level;*
- *a life of service to the greater good of humanity;*
- *a life of non-violence.*

---

[25] See Appendices for an 'About The Author' section.

All of this was pursued as a spiritual path, and through his unrelenting pursuit of truth and service, and therefore justice, this inevitably led him into what we would call political activity (or public life), in order to attempt to right the obvious wrongs and injustices he saw around him.

Gandhi was without question an extra-ordinary man. His influence for the good of humanity was perhaps as great as any other person of the 20th century. One of his strongest desires was to see communities where people were living simple, sustainable lives, based on self-reliance and a pursuit of physical and spiritual health.

Gandhi remains a powerful influence and inspiration to many people. I commend all readers to understand the importance of simplifying one's life and limiting the influences of consumerism, TV and the media, as this is a simple and powerful way that we as individuals can move towards a more ecologically sustainable life.

If we can live a life of service for the greater good then we are really getting somewhere – whether its selling 'good' products or services (i.e. that contribute to creating genuine wisdom, health and/or sustainability), developing ethical financial and investment strategies, providing positive education, working in the public or community sector or growing organic food.

Eating more raw is important – but there's a lot more for us to sort out than diet. Unless we face up to that and start making equally fundamental changes in other areas of our lives, we are going to be forced to deal with our lack of responsibility further down the line, and it will not be fun. At least that's what my experiments with the truth tell me.

Please start your researches now beyond just health, and take actions to improve the sustainability and the positive effects of your life in as many areas as you can. Your work is one of your most important effects in the world. Are you working for health and sustainability or are you working against them? Look at how so many people involved in the natural health and ecological worlds have already changed their life and work, and are still doing it, and how much better they feel for doing it ...You can do it too.

"Be the Change you want to see in the world." M.K.Gandhi

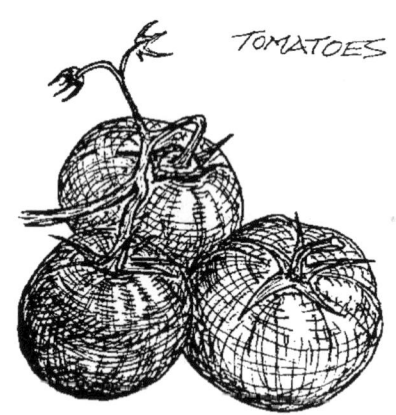

Working With Nature: The Route to Personal & Planetary Health

The combination of a wider understanding of health creating nutrition and sustainable living gives us a serious yet playful, utterly democratic route to creating individual and community health, greater freedom and much greater self-reliance and self-confidence.

The environment, relationships and life we create around us all come through our thoughts and values, and the actions that follow them. If we see, feel or understand this, then we start to sense how a more sustainable lifestyle can be created.

At the moment we often place the responsibility for sustainability and health outside ourselves; with the government, doctors, drug companies and the health service. At their current level of thinking, government policy and the medical establishment will *never* create health. Because they are focused on illness, not health – they maintain a dependency culture that is self-justifying, which accepts and believes that high levels of sickness are 'normal'.

Equally, while unhealthy foods are very costly for our health, they are profitable for the drug and medical industry, and for the food processing industry, and their shareholders. I'm not sure that many people knowingly make others sick for profit – generally it is a cycle that our clever but unwise society is locked into because we don't know any better, with profit being a higher political priority than creating real health. We don't learn about health from nature, because as a modern, developed, scientific society we tend to think we know better than nature. We observe nature on TV endlessly, or read about it, but most of us simply don't 'know' or experience it anymore, because our own nature has become so distorted and separated from nature – including by eating 'food' that is an industrial product, with not an ounce of nature left in it.

Some people do think there is more to our poor state of human and planetary health than just chance. Health and freedom have a close relationship. If someone loses their health they often lose their freedom. How would that feel to you? Think about it. A population that lives in fear of sickness, chronic illness and death is not a free society. Fear leads to a dependency on earning money to pay for health insurance, medical care and the distractions needed to suppress or hide the fear, or feed the addictions. A population that is 'dumbed down' with heavy and addictive foods may be easier to manipulate and exploit. So I've heard some people say in a jokey way "You aren't going to eat more of that conspiracy food are you?".

For those who are into conspiracy theories, look at the relationship between food, health and freedom – or rather food, illness and loss of freedom - you might just find one of the biggest potential conspiracies going, if that's what you're looking for. But *I suggest that the key thing is to be part of a positive, health creating conspiracy, and start with yourself*, as it's the only place you can start. Whatever you think, the point is that if you want health you have to create it for yourself. And we can all achieve improved health once we understand the nature of health.

In creating individual and community health we break the dependency culture that is justified and maintained by people's understandable fears of various chronic conditions of ill-health, which typically grows as people get older. We can transform an economy that profits (massively) from ill-health and the products that create chronic illness, to an economy and culture which profits from health – which may be starting already with growing a 'sub-economy' and 'sub-culture' of health creation. We can become more able and confident in meeting our own needs, and move ourselves closer to a vision of health and sustainability in the process.

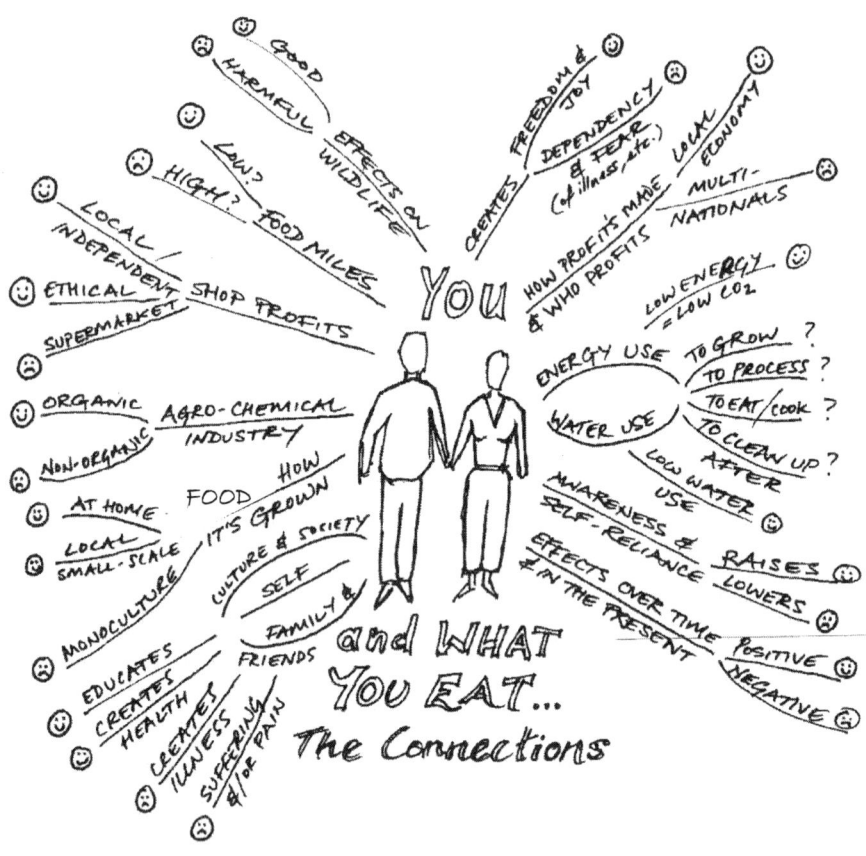

The Big Challenge to Us as Individuals and the World

The Creative Margins

For the pioneering and admirable, yet currently small but growing worlds of health creation, raw food and permaculture, as a positive challenge, I want to be clear that from both an entirely 'rational' logical perspective and a deep feeling, gut-level instinct:

a) if properly rooted in an understanding of natural health creation and food vitality, *every healthy living advocate and raw fooder in the world should be growing at least some of their own food, using a permaculture approach*;

- If you are a healthy living advocate or raw fooder, you need to contemplate this deeply, **and act on it** from a whole health creating perspective;

b) if fully and properly rooted in the attitudes and principles of permaculture and ecology, including the ecology of health, then *every permaculturalist in the world should be designing and implementing health creating lifestyles, with that normally including 50% or more raw, largely home or locally grown*;

- If you are a permaculturalist, you need to contemplate this deeply, **and act on it** from a permaculture design and action perspective.

This perspective needs to widely understood and implemented. A culture, *or a growing sub-culture*, that adopts or adapts this goal at its core will be the first to have an all-encompassing vision of whole health at its heart.

The Stuck and Stagnant Mainstream

For the mainstream, the first step is to accept the following - there is no hope whatsoever, in any way at all, that the *current* dominant medical/pharmaceutical paradigm, and all the institutional 'health' (sic) systems that support them, can achieve *anything at all* to a) improve health *on any significant scale*, or b) reduce the *massive and steadily growing* social and financial costs of widespread chronic ill-health.

Practitioners and administrators, politicians, and anyone working in the 'health' system have to understand that *the only hope* for an improvement in the situation, is a *radical change* in thinking, understanding and practice i.e. change at the root level.

Significant levels of health can be achieved – massive levels of illness reduction can be achieved – only if and when a fundamentally different approach is adopted. This can be done on an individual or family level, or on the level of a group, community or culture.

However, *this can only be achieved if it is based in an understanding of the natural processes of health creation, and the natural processes of maintenance and support of health. The following sections explain how this can be achieved, at any level.*

PART 4: THE STRATEGY - THRIVE BY MEETING YOUR NEEDS

SUSTAINABLE LIVING MEANS MEETING YOUR HEALTHY NEEDS

In developing our western ideas about our psychological *needs* and psychological *health*, the fundamental theory and practices of psychology were *not* based on studying people who were *healthy*, but were based on studying people who suffered disturbed behaviour or mental illness.[26] However, the humanistic psychologist Abraham Maslow studied *healthy, fully functional individuals*, to reveal people's needs in this healthy state. Maslow's picture of needs therefore differs considerably from virtually all preceding psychological theory and practice that studied only the sick. His description of healthy human needs is summarised as follows:

Maslow's Needs Hierarchy

Physiological Needs:
Biological needs for oxygen, food,
water and suitable body temperature.
Without these strongest needs met we die.

Safety Needs:
Children experience these fairly continually, whilst
adults experience these needs in periods of disruption.

Love, Affection and Belongingness Needs:
Needs to avoid loneliness and alienation, needs to connect with
others and needs to give and receive love, affection and belonging.

Esteem Needs:
Self-respect and respect from others, required for confidence in our thinking,
decisions and actions. Without these, people feel inferior, weak, helpless and worthless.

Self-Actualisation / Fulfillment:
This is the individual achieving what she or he was born to do - fulfilling a 'calling', following your path. Without this the person is restless and something is just not right with the world.

Our current culture leaves many of these healthy needs unmet. What kind of individuals, families, communities and society will we have when we prioritize these needs, and use the economy intelligently to meet these needs? What good reason is there not to aim for this now? Do we deserve these things for ourselves and our children? How can you start to gradually meet these needs more fully?

---

[26] It is worth pondering for a moment about how things might change if our medical research studied physical health and health creation much more than they studied illness and disease.

It makes complete sense to look for sustainable ways to meet these needs. Our uniquely sophisticated body, brain and consciousness emerged from a raw, evolutionary recipe that met all our needs, and which enabled our unique human consciousness to emerge. Generally what we eat now is very different from that evolutionary recipe.

To what extent does our current diet meet our physiological-biological-neurological needs for the optimum health of our mind-body-consciousness system? Can we have any realistic idea of our genuine needs unless we actually experience different diets and lifestyles? How do our lifestyles and living environments affect our hierarchy of needs?

As both Einstein and Buddha said, genuine knowledge comes only from experience. Anything else is simply ideas in our head, that creates the illusion of knowing based on 'ideas about' something rather than genuine experience. So, only when *you experience* some degree of an 'eat more raw' lifestyle will you actually know its effects – although you may of course have a head full of 'ideas about' its effects. Only when you try it over a long enough period of time, in a well-informed way, will you ever *know the effects on your needs over time*, and will you ever *find out if your ideas are right* or misinformed. The same is true of sustainable living.

Through direct experience I know that an 'eat more raw' lifestyle meets more of my needs. It is becoming more known in our society and generates interest, although some people do still see it as odd (which I find weird because it just feels so natural to me!). And for the many that have tried it, this is not theory – they have tried it, so they now know. Because my choices are based on *good information, personal experience* and a *strong feeling* of my needs being met, I feel free and confident about my choices. I've seen again and again that as people shift to eating more raw, health-creating foods, and shift to more sustainable living, people start to notice, and as a result the economy and society change, little-by-little.

Combining natural health and sustainable living offers many benefits and we cannot really achieve one without the other, and here's why:

- the optimum conditions for creating health of any living organism depend on the health of the whole living system of the Earth
- the optimum conditions for creating health of any person depends on the health of the society and living systems of the Earth
- all living things are born with the natural right, innate expectation and capacity to experience real health

Sustainable living means enjoying a balanced health creating diet, a fulfilling lifestyle and designing an efficient, beautiful home. On a wider level it means creating eco-neighbourhoods, eco-schools, ecovillages and eco-cities, within healthy bioregions, with vibrant economies and a culture of health and creativity. Think about the effects on the global ecosystem and local ecosystems if we changed from eating foods that create degraded environments, and instead consciously ate healthy foods and crops which we produced in ways that only enhance biodiversity, soil quality and ecosystems health.

Fully sustainable living is healthy living and vice versa – this is real health on a whole system level. It means sustainable/healthy work, sustainable/healthy homes and sustainable/healthy leisure, and in practice this also means all the following:

- Sust'n'healthy energy use: high efficiency, reduced demand, sustainable/renewable supply
- Sust'n'healthy buildings and construction: transformed existing buildings through sustainable/healthy retrofit, and sustainable/healthy new build
- Sust'n'healthy resource/materials use and management: reduce, re-use, recycle, dematerialization, substituting non-toxic low impact services and products for high impact ones, circular resource cycles, etc
- Sust'n'healthy diets and food systems: organic, local/bioregional, reduced packaging, energy inputs and food miles, etc
- Sust'n'healthy access and mobility: reduced travel, use of local facilities and resources, most sustainable transport options, etc

Everyone can make changes in these areas, some big changes, some smaller. It also requires:
- Education for sustainability/health: environmental and development education, education for creativity and effectiveness, within sustainable/healthy eco-schools, colleges and universities, teaching people (staff as much as students!) to live and work sustainably
- Sustainable health creation: learning to create health, in healthy sustainable buildings
- Sustainable/healthy livelihoods and consumption: sustainable/healthy consumption is important, *and* sustainable/healthy work / livelihoods is equally important – *only* if our *work* is *truly* creating genuine health and sustainability is our biggest contribution to the economy adding to the solutions, rather than the problems.

If you understand how you understand, you can use that insight to help create environments and lifestyles that naturally generate health and sustainability. This may mean creating some mental image or feeling for how things can change. It may mean focusing on your body to let it tell your mind which foods are health creating foods – feeling different tastes in your mouth and *the feeling of foods within your body*. It means taking responsibility for your patterns of thinking and values, and for your systems of growing or buying food, systems of gaining a living, and your involvement with other people, so that these are in harmony.

A harmonious, compassionate way of life is often very powerful when you let go of the endless rationalizing, and at its most beautiful when there is no busy, busy thinking. Conflict and friction can dissolve when there is no need to understand or control, because inner trust and knowing create inner peace, clear direction and harmonious action. Amazing things can happen when we allow nature's innate intelligence (which is part of all of us) to create better levels of health for us, which is all it ever really wants to do.

- Visualise yourself living in a more naturally healthy and sustainable way. Or write a story about how you create health in your life in the future.
- What would feeling naturally healthy feel like? Imagine and describe or illustrate that in whatever way suits you. Sing about it if you like!

This philosophy of *working with nature* allows your thinking to flow into action because there is an inner knowing that is in accord with principles of healthy, sustainable living. In this way an inner feeling of trust is there which guides your thoughts and actions without the mind jabbering away, trying to control everything.

In many ways, this is the *Tao of Health* – it offers three keys to sustainable health:
- UNDERSTANDING / KNOWING THE NATURE OF UNDERSTANDING
- UNDERSTANDING / KNOWING THE NATURE OF HEALTH
- UNDERSTANDING / KNOWING THE NATURE OF NATURE

REAL HEALTH

For complete, holistic health and wellbeing, for the individual, our culture (people in general) and the world's ecosystems, we have to create real health in both our internal ecosystems and our external ecosystems, which is a two stage process:

    a)   cleansing, detoxifying and purifying

    b)   creating and maintaining a healthy organism, and health-creating systems

In both these stages, appropriate 'nutrition' is key to a multi-dimensional health creating process, and cannot be ignored, whether it is nutrition for an organism or for an ecosystem.

We need to take a problem-solution-strategy approach:
- Problem – disease creating diet and lifestyle
- Solution – health creating diet and lifestyle
- Strategy – adopt eat more raw lifestyle and holistic health creating lifestyle (including work), as part of developing a sustainable, positive and fulfilling lifestyle

Dimensions of the eat more raw lifestyle:
- EMR lifestyle as a personal development pathway
- EMR lifestyle as a process of cultural evolution and social change
- EMR lifestyle as a strand of health and environmental activism, or philosophy
- EMR lifestyle for vibrant health, clear mind, changed awareness and understanding

---

If you do not feel drawn to try a high percentage raw diet, at least think about the beneficial impacts of eating more raw foods. Think about the impacts in the wider world and in your own life. Have the courage to cut back your wheat, meat and dairy for a week, fortnight or month and see what the experiment brings. [27] Try a mainly raw week or month here and there, fruit only mornings, a regular juice day or some high quality super foods. Give yourself the chance to *know for yourself from experience*, and discover the difference between your ideas of how it would be and the reality. Flexibility and adaptability in diet and lifestyle can only help you increase your freedom and independence, your choices and self-reliance. Give it a try.

---

[27] See the booklet *Grain Damage*, Foodnsport Press (2005) by Dr Douglas Graham for a full run down on the environmental and health related effects of a high-wheat diet – referenced in Appendices section.

KNOWLEDGE AS THE FRUIT OF EXTENDED OBSERVATION & EXPERIENCE

What I eat has changed my life significantly, with several of my 'reality tunnels' blown apart since starting to explore different diets and lifestyles. I ate an omnivorous diet (with lots of meat) for the first 26 years of my life, and was then vegetarian and a non-evangelical vegan, for 3 years each (i.e. I just got on and did it). Then I was raw vegan for 11 years. All in all, I've been all or high raw consistently since autumn '94. For about 10 years I was fairly active within the raw food movement, and have known a number of the active advocates and educators in the raw movement, and have observed many people following various all or mainly raw diets. I have done this: while working in the mainstream as a sustainability consultants; while living in a raw eco-community off-grid (i.e. with no electrical appliances) on a Spanish hillside with my dwelling being a large ex-army tent; as a single man; as a father in a family situation; and then as a single parent 3-days a week. So my knowledge is based on extended observation and considerable experience of a broad variety of different situations.

So, to me, a high percentage raw food diet includes a variety of options:

- The eclectic 'raw + super-foods' approach promoted by Dave Wolfe, Shazzie, Kate Wood, Mike Nash and many others
- Robert Hart's 'R70 forest garden diet' (70% raw fruit, 'sallets' and nuts/seeds)[28]
- A 'living foods' diet as promoted by Dr Brian Clements, Elaine Bruce and others
- A natural hygiene lifestyle promoted by Dave Klein, Dr Douglas Graham, Professor Rozalind Gruben and many others
- Eating only or mainly fruit (called 'fruitarian' although technically called 'frugivorous')
- Sibila's nature-guided, simple and intuitive and spiritual approach (see later sections)
- Dr Gabriel Cousen's individualized and person specific approach to nutritional needs
- Tony Wright's extraordinary work on neurologically & reproductively regenerative nutrition
- A nutrient-dense 'funky raw' lifestyle and approach to raising 'radiant children'

There is also the 'instincto' philosophy, which is quite distinct from the vast majority of the all / mainly raw movement. This philosophy suggests we tap into our instincts to determine what and when we want to eat, and how much, particularly through our sense of smell before eating and our sense of taste whilst we eat. There is value in this, and vegetarian or vegan instincto's who I have come across seem very balanced and healthy people. However, much of this movement includes raw meat and fish eating as part of the diet. The few raw meat / fish eating instincto's I have met have generally appeared to me less healthy and balanced (psychologically and physiologically), so this is not something I or mainstream raw food advocates recommend. From my limited experience of this movement, instincto kitchens have an underlying repulsive smell, and as far as I can tell there seem to be real dangers in consistently eating raw meat, although

---

[28] Robert Hart was a wonderful gentleman whose ideas on forest gardening have had a major impact on the British permaculture movement – in particular through his books *Forest Gardening*, Green Earth books (1996) and *Beyond the Forest Garden*, Gaia Books (1996).

possibly this depends on the quantity and quality. To my knowledge this small, mainly French movement, is the only group that promotes raw meat eating. Some limit themselves to eating raw fish. The founder Guy Claude Berger served a term in prison for his other unsavoury ideas and habits that were part of his libertarian philosophy, not related to his diet. His wife died of bowel cancer, having followed this diet for many years as I understand it.

Daniel Vitalis has moved from raw vegan to a 'wild diet', and focuses on 'natural foods', and 'indigenous nutrition'. To me his changing position makes sense in terms of a survivalist perspective, and in many practical ways - but not from an evolutionary or optimum health perspective compared with Tony Wright, whose focus is on the complex biochemistry of certain food groups, and the awesome sophistication of evolutionary bio-molecular engineering.

The results and benefits of the various vegan and vegetarian approaches to a high raw diet vary from person to person, with some having better results than others. In my experience of observing others on a fruitarian path, this diet seems not to suit our culture and the food quality that is generally available (i.e. demineralized, hybridized, high-sugar, low-mineral fruits, with massive food miles), except perhaps in short bursts. It is highly idealistic and very attractive in many ways - however it is likely to be less grounded and balanced, particularly for those of us living in the 'normal' world – although in a rich and diverse tropical forest garden, if makes plenty of sense. Some of those that I've known who have followed this approach for a long period have *not* been pictures of health at all - whilst a few are fantastic examples of health.

The focus *in this book* is what is *relevant and accessible to the majority* - that is what is important for creating the greatest cumulative health benefit. For most people experimenting with different levels of raw in their diet, up to about 75% fruit seems fine (if it's ripe and not overly hybridized – and ideally mainly grown locally/regionally). Beyond that, for most people, greens in particular and certain essential fats are vital for gaining a full range of minerals which are vital for body and brain health, and difficult to gain from many fruits, particularly the limited and expensive range of often unripe fruit that is on offer from supermarkets.

In my experience different approaches are good to try, you learn from them, and they can all have benefits. In the longer term a balanced fruit and veg approach, with simple (simply delicious!) meals is normally the best to settle into, with the fruit-veg balance varied to the season and climate you live in, as well as your activity levels and personality, and ensuring a good level of nutrient density is important. Intuitively and logically this kind of diet is a 'more natural diet' for us. Much of this book aims to show why this is the case.

Generally the key flexible guidelines in raw food nutrition *for adults* include:

- sensible food combining – see food combining chart in *Part Two: The Practicalities*;
- eating a reasonably low protein but *nutrient-dense diet* i.e. rich in minerals, vitamins and EFAs (essential fatty acids);
- eating the highest quality fats from vegetable / seed / fruit sources;
- a reasonable balance of fruits, vegetables and really *good quality greens*.

If you get these 4 parts of your diet right, then in some ways the rest doesn't matter!

Part Five of this book addresses – *The Practicalities* - all these issues in more detail, as well as covering the most balanced approach for children.

NATURE AS YOUR GUIDE TO HEALTH

So what guidelines are there on how nature works as a health-creating system?

Sustainability and permaculture are about designing and creating ecologically sustainable, efficient and productive systems and about "designing sustainable lifestyles"[29]. So as sustainability and health are essentially interchangeable and interdependent, we can equally use permaculture to design and create healthy systems and healthy lifestyles.

This represents consistency in our whole system approach to health and sustainability, as it means we are looking at the ecology of our own 'natural' mind-body-spirit system (our internal ecology) as well as the ecology of the external environment – and the interconnected relationships and interactions between these inner and outer worlds. *We can design these inner and outer dimensions to be positive and health creating.*

All life, including human life, soil, woodland and forest life, is a *regenerative, health building process*, provided it has the environment, nutrition and healthy immune system to create this. Nature naturally creates health – that is its primary interest and basic objective. Physiology and anatomy *always* tells us every creature's nutritional needs for health - and if those needs are met, whilst living in a healthy environment, health will be the natural outcome.

Our body is a flowing mass of interconnected health-sustaining, health-creating processes - given the chance it *always* regenerates itself naturally. What we eat is a key factor in shaping how and with what this happens. We all know "you are what you eat". Most of our body is water, and over 95% of our cells are replaced within one year, with virtually every cell in our body replaced in 7 years – we are literally a different person.[30]

To be healthy we need to regenerate our cells with the best possible materials, fuels and lubricants. Raw foods encourage the body's healing and regenerative processes by working with nature, whilst many common processed foods hinder the body's healing and regenerative process – they work against nature. Raw foods are rich in vital water, vitamins and minerals, are nutrient-dense, provide the highest quality fats, and naturally help shift toxins out of the body. While many cooked and processed foods are dehydrated or dehydrating, demineralised, nutrient-poor and provide the worst quality of corrupted fats, bringing more toxins into the body, and actively inhibiting the body's ability to shift the junk out.

Also, drinking good quality water really helps create health and vitality, keeping us hydrated and flushing unwanted toxins from our cells, through the inter-cellular fluid. So, even as an adult, your body is a flow of interconnected processes, not an unchanging solid object.

The natural way our digestive system works means that *all* nutrition passes into our body in liquid form through the walls of the digestive system. Liquid rich whole raw organic plant foods such as fruits, greens, salad leaves and vegetables are the best vehicles for transporting these essential life giving, health-creating minerals, vitamins and enzymes into our body. They require less work for the body to take in that nutrition. And they represent a flow of life giving energy.

---

[29] This is the British permaculture teacher Stephen Nutt's simple and useful definition of permaculture.

[30] Dr Deepak Chopra, *Ageless Body, Timeless Mind*, Random House Audiobooks (1990).

To understand how diet and lifestyle can create health you need to: a) generate a vision of how your body works as a flowing system of inter-connected processes, a cleansing, healing river of life, a health creating process; b) feel your body's innate ability and desire to create and maintain health; c) sense how to work with nature to create that health.

Some basic facts about the nutritional nature of foods are very useful to know. *Firstly*, long term raw fooder, ex-Olympic trampolinist, and health adviser to top athletes Dr Doug Graham highlights the accepted nutritional facts about basic food groups:

- Fresh raw FRUITS are the *very best* source of VITAMINS and the second best source of minerals.
- Fresh raw VEGETABLES (particularly greens) are the *very best* source of MINERALS and the second best source of vitamins.

Remember these facts above! They are vital ... literally.

So eating plenty of fresh raw fruit, greens and vegetables *ensures* your diet is well supplied from the very best sources of vitamins and minerals. It's that simple. 'Five portions a day' is better than none, and will improve most people's health – and if you go well beyond 5 a day, making sure the portions are all / mainly raw, you'll gain *much greater* health benefits. You don't need expensive pills and potions to get the best – you simply have to grow or buy nature's vitamin and mineral packages - they're called fruits, vegetables, nuts and seeds.

Raw foods contain plenty of purified water as well as all its nutrients, so they are great body cleansers. Meanwhile the chlorophyll that is in green leafy vegetables is a wonderful healer and rebuilder of the body. It's a fascinating fact that chlorophyll is essentially identical in structure to the hemoglobin in our blood – except that hemoglobin centres on an iron molecule, whilst it's a magnesium molecule for chlorophyll.

A *second key fact*, emphasized by many, is that green leafy vegetables are the best foods for obtaining the proteins we need to build and maintain our body. So Popeye was right after all - better to get it fresh and raw than out of a can though! Greens are the best protein builders because they contain the essential amino acids, minerals and vitamins that enable the body to build the proteins it needs – this is explained in more detail in the FAQ section later (see 'the Protein Question'). Green leaves are also the most alkaline foods, which is very important and beneficial – and is explained later in the Acid-Alkaline Balance section.

So fruits and vegetables are the very best sources for the vitamins, minerals and sugars we need. And well stored seeds and nuts, as well as avocados and other fatty fruits, are the best sources for the fats we need, with organic raw coconut oil being the 'queen of fats', whilst cool-stored organic cold pressed flax and hemp oils are excellent too (as is Udo's Choice oil blend). Sprouted pulses and seeds, such as alfalfa, chickpeas, green lentils, mung and so on are also packed with vital proteins, enzymes, vitamins and minerals. So by making sure we have an appropriate balance of these nutrient rich foods in their natural raw state, we can meet all our body's essential needs with ease. So *if the flow of processes that your body is made up is a flow of health-creating foods, it will naturally create health* - you won't have to work for it.

Even our brain cells depend on flows and maintenance processes. For example, DHA (Docosahexaenoic acid), an omega-3 fatty acid, is known to be essential for growth and development of brain function in infants and children, and also for maintaining proper brain function in adults. Adequate dietary DHA improves learning ability, whilst DHA deficiencies seem to impair learning and raise the risk of depression and Alzheimer's. DHA is taken up by the brain in preference to other fatty acids and the use of DHA in the brain appears to be fast.[31]

It is also worth noting that some plants naturally have particularly beneficial effects. So particularly powerful foods can be integrated into the ecology of any dietary system. These might include: *Ginkgo biloba* leaves for their brain and circulation improving qualities; *Hippophae rhamnoides/salicifolia* (Seabuckthorn) for its small, nutrient-packed fruits that are being researched for use against cancer; Goji berries (*Lycium barbarum*) are also very nutrient rich – and surprisingly easy to grow in many climates; and St Johns wort (*Hypericum*) for its beneficial effects on the brain, which when combined with *Passiflora* makes an excellent 'happy tea' mix. Numerous superfoods are also available, with DHA supplements (e.g. O-Mega-Zen produced by NuTru), ionic zinc supplements, ionic trace minerals (e.g. from Marine Minerals) and a variety of other products worthy of consideration.

It is important to *recognize the extraordinary diversity of nutrients in the plant kingdom*. Almost anything and everything imaginable is available in the plant kingdom, including around 70,000 known edible plants, as well as medicinal plants. In the next 10 years or so we'll see many more people *design nutrient rich mixed ecologies, consciously planted and grown to supply a nutrient rich diet - this is an emerging future – it is* **Nutrition Gardening**.

From an ecological perspective, we can also sense how matter and energy *flow* through us. Matter in some forms creates health, whilst in other forms it creates sickness. Some forms of matter generate energy in our body, whilst other forms use more energy in the body than they create. So by seeing foods as flows of matter and energy, you can see or feel the many relationships matter and energy have with both inner and outer health. Then you can sense how those relationships can be used to create and support personal and ecological health.

After all, which contains more of the energy of life, nature, planet earth, Gaia, Goddess, God - a crisp apple or fresh green salad, or chips, a Big Mac or sausage?

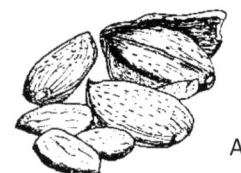
Almonds

If your foods contain no life force (or Tao) then what other forces do they contain instead? Think about it!

If you are an environmentalist, ethical consumer, 'green' or you deeply respect the life's sacredness, nature or Gaia, God, or creation, if you are a vegetarian or vegan, then you may find that eating more raw is wholly in line with your ethics and values, and may take them further, helping you build your bodily 'temple' from natural, health giving materials. Health can only help you achieve more of what you are called to achieve through the life choices you make.

---

[31] DHA is available as a supplement, a very beneficial form is derived from algae oil. See www.veganesentials.com – look for NuTru O-Mega-Zen DHA capsules. See the work of Prof M A Crawford for the key role of Omega-3's in neurological health and their deficiency in many standard western diets.

SUSTAINABLE LIVING, HEALTH AND PERMACULTURE

Permaculture is both an ethical ecological design system and a movement concerned with the impacts of the ways in which we live our lives. Its object is to find practical ways of transforming our lifestyle impacts from negative to positive - environmentally, socially and economically. It has been described as applied common sense, and the most useful of 'green' ideas. It is a solutions-oriented system of lifestyle and landscape design and a set of tools and techniques for creating sustainable lifestyles and sustainable human habitats.

"Permaculture provides positive solutions for us all, to create environmentally sustainable, harmonious and abundant ways of living" – Aranya, source: www.learnpermaculture.com

The term 'permaculture' comes from combining the ideas of permanent agriculture (including horticulture and silviculture) and permanent culture.

"Permaculture is the conscious design and maintenance of agriculturally productive ecosystems which have the diversity, stability and resilience of natural ecosystems. It is the harmonious integration of landscape and people providing their food, energy, shelter, and other material and non-material needs in a sustainable way..."
Bill Mollison, *Permaculture: A Designers' Manual*, Tagari Press (1988).

As stated already, health and sustainability are essentially the same processes, one within the person (or organism), the other within the environment. Permaculture is an evolving set of ideas, practices and lifestyles that provides us with a practical set of tools to move us towards sustainable living – these tools are also fantastically useful when the focus is health creation.

This book explains how permaculture thinking can also be used to design and create naturally healthy lifestyles - which is an essential aspect of sustainability to me. Diet, food and nutrition are important parts of any culture and have to be core concerns for a sustainable culture. A truly sustainable culture must be a naturally healthy culture – so we need some coherent and robust models of health creation to help us achieve this.

Permaculture was well designed to be beyond the ownership of any person by Bill Mollison, with David Holmgren – this is one of its strengths. Its ethics and principles are applied differently by different people – for example, there are now many vegan permaculture systems, as well as permaculture systems applied to organic mixed farms and gardens. So don't think that permaculture is any one way of doing things – it can be an art or science, a mental technology or spiritually based philosophy, or a mix of these - so long as it gets results where its three core ethics meet.

Fundamentally it is a way of thinking and living that is about 'designing sustainable lifestyles', and putting solutions into action. It has three core ethics:

EARTH CARE   PEOPLE CARE   FAIR SHARE

These three ethics provide a good starting point for considering how to meet our needs in ways that naturally create sustainable health. After considering these core ethics, we will look at six permaculture design principles, and how they are relevant to health, nutrition and diet.

EARTH CARE: ECOLOGICAL SUSTAINABILITY

Earth Care - the optimum conditions for creating health of any living organism depend on the health of the living systems of the Earth.

In most habitable climates nature will create a forest if it is left alone - Ecology calls this the 'climax ecosystem'. These are generally the most productive land-based ecosystems in terms of biodiversity (variety and quantity of species) and plant biomass, and the most sophisticated and productive in terms of complex biochemistry. Woodlands and forests are stable, and create and maintain soil fertility through a vast range of beneficial and productive relationships between trees and other plants, animals, insects, bacteria, fungi, worms, soil and so on. If all the elements in the system are healthy and interacting properly with each other then we have complete system health.

For me, Earth Care means a general intention of care for all the Earth's living creatures, which are part of the Earth's web of life. So I prefer a vegetarian or vegan lifestyle, and food producing habitats that supply the needs of both humans and wildlife.

While growing huge quantities of wheat (even for organic wholemeal bread or pasta) means mono-cultural arable deserts, involving massive energy and agro-chemical use. The Romans extended the Sahara significantly because north Africa was their wheat growing belt (even without using agrochemicals and heavy agricultural machinery). To grow wheat 'successfully' we mimic its natural environment (i.e. semi-desert) and create, maintain and expand man-made semi-desert landscapes all around the world – much of it for animal fodder - these are not biodiverse or stable environments. To me this is not an ideal strategy for Earth Care or sustainability!

In contrast, fruit grows on trees, and root crops, tubers, squashes, legumes and salads can be grown as part of a permaculture forest garden or local market garden, small farm and agroforestry systems, with less energy inputs and creating a diverse and stable habitat. Permaculture systems actively create soil health, and diverse interacting regenerative plant ecologies. Forest gardening and agro-forestry can maximise care for the earth and all its inhabitants, as they are based on creating highly productive, diverse and stable forest and woodland ecosystems. They are ideal for a high percentage raw diet, and for supplying many other needs such as timber and fibres. That's what I call Earth Care!

Obviously, the essential task of Earth Care is to create healthy ecoystems, including *healthy organisms* and processes within those ecosystems and healthy relationships between them.

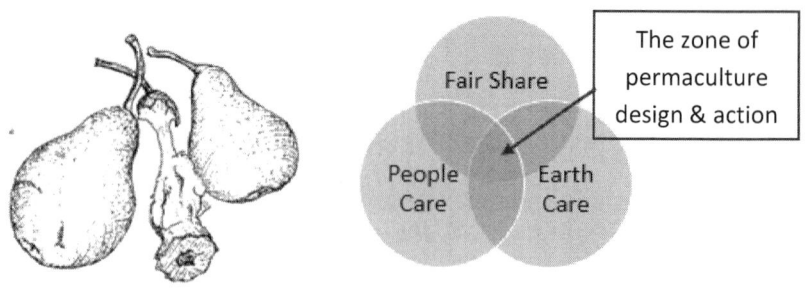

PEOPLE CARE: MEETING HUMAN NEEDS

People Care – the optimum conditions for creating health of any person depends on the health of the society and living systems of the Earth, and vice versa.

People Care is about meeting our many and diverse needs, as individuals and groups, because *we need to care for ourselves as part of the Earth*. Ecological thinking and sustainable living can meet these needs: physical, security, love, affection, belongingness, esteem and our needs for fulfillment in life – the healthy needs as identified by Abraham Maslow. So to me, *to maximise People Care, we need to seek and create vibrant health in people* – physical, mental, emotional and spiritual – as individuals and cultures.

Raw foods cleanse the body's systems, increase alkalinity (see later section on acid / alkaline balance), boost the immune system and thereby support health and healing. A healthier lifestyle and diet also reduces the chance of friends and family suffering as a result of a loved-one's illness. So acting to reduce the 'web of suffering' by living a health-creating lifestyle is something excellent People Care. Even if I alone take responsibility for my own health, that helps avoid the worry and emotional pain others might experience if I became ill – which is caring for those who care for me. Therefore, *creating health is at the heart of People Care*, and in many ways an 'eat more raw' lifestyle is an extremely powerful way of living this ethic.

FAIR SHARE: EQUITY IN CHOICE, AND SHARING SURPLUS

(Sometimes termed 'Resources for Need, not Greed')

Fair Share – in general living things are born with the natural right, expectation and capacity to experience real health.

This is about fair resource consumption and sharing surpluses. For me, Fair Share means aiming for everyone and everything having its basic needs met, and is also about:

1. Aiming to make sure that our lifestyle only uses our fair share of planetary resources – less than a third of resource impacts of a typical western diet and lifestyle.
2. Actively avoiding exploitation of humans or animals, plants, soils, landscape or habitats.
3. Sharing our surpluses.

David Wolfe points out that nature has provided raw plant foods as *by far* the most naturally abundant foods on the planet because this is an efficient, effective system that really works. That's why so much life depends and thrives on them. *Abundance* means the chance of fair shares for all. Meanwhile industrial animal farming creates scarcity because it is so resource hungry, in terms of land, water, energy, animal fodder and so on.

All life should have its fair share of resources. An *eat more raw* lifestyle, catered for by forest gardening, agroforestry, organic horticulture and permaculture can meet all our physical needs. This is a great vision for a fair and equitable way of meeting human needs through ecologically positive and sustainable food growing systems that leaves more land for biodiverse nature, using ecologically and energy efficient, healthy and accessible ways to feed ourselves, whilst also catering for the needs of so many other living things.

To summarise, in practice, an eat more raw lifestyle and permaculture are about:

- *Solutions* that *combine* Earth Care, People Care and Fair Shares;
- *Observing* over time, to see, feel and experience the nature of nature, the nature of health creation, and to understand our web of effects in our immediate and wider world;
- *Taking action* to ensure our web of effects is positive as possible in ecological and health terms, for ourselves and the outer world.
- *Developing positive, healthy and beneficial relationships* between the elements and activities of our life, in our living and built environment.

ATTITUDE PRINCIPLES AND THEIR BENEFITS TO DIET AND HEALTH

Bill Mollison and David Holmgren's early work, as the founders of Permaculture, led to the following six principles emerging as powerful guides to ecological and healthy thinking. They are ecological truisms which can be used to design and live a healthy and sustainable life.

WORK WITH NATURE, NOT AGAINST IT

This principle was the inspiration for this book and is the fundamental basis of my understanding of health and sustainability. Contemplate this principle for a minute, an hour, a day or a year - it may change your life. Its simplicity oozes truth and wisdom. It recognizes that nature knows best when it comes to creating both health and productive, diverse sustainable living systems. From one perspective nature is health – *with the right conditions nature always naturally manifests health. So, if we create those conditions or get close to them, we can know what creates health* - and that involves working with nature.

Looking into human evolution is one way to get a sense of what is natural to us. But, our theories of human evolution are based on a lot of guess work because so little evidence of early human and pre-human life has been found. In reality, tiny snippets of a vast puzzle are all we have. However, some evidence is very solid - anatomically and physiologically humans are categorized as 'great apes', and the 'highest' of the higher primates, in our primate family tree. This tells us a lot about our evolution, and our evolutionary diet. All other 'great apes' evolved in and still live in tropical forests, indicating that early humans also developed in the forests. This is consistent with known facts about historical climate change that shrank the early 'humans' tropical forest home, pushing us out onto the expanded savannah. [32]

We adapted to the savannah, and later still to a huge range of historical and modern living conditions, many of which are bizarre in evolutionary terms. However, tropical forest dwelling was certainly our natural evolutionary home, and gave us our evolutionary diet – this has major implications for understanding our 'natural' diet, to help us live in healthy ways.

---

[32] Archeologists will never find skeletons of our forest dwelling ancestors as tropical forest ecosystems, break down all bodies and skeletons quickly and efficiently - archeologists are not ecologists so they don't think about such obvious factors. Thus they think humans developed on the savannahs, because that's the only skeleton evidence they've found – this is understandable, but not clever or logical, and certainly not scientific.

Standard anatomical and zoological science helps us understand what 'natural' means for us. Dennis Nelson's great little book *Maximizing Your Nutrition* notes the five basic zoological categories of Animals, based on their anatomy and physiology, and *describes the accepted scientific perspective that every animal's body-type indicates very clearly how it is specialized in a) eating particular foods, and b) a particular environment:*[33] *In other words, physiology and anatomy tell us the natural diet and natural environment of all creatures ... including humans.*

- *Carnivores:* with claws, large canine teeth, beaks or incredibly strong jaws for tearing skin and flesh, with short digestive systems, high acidity digestive system to kill meat-related bacteria and parasites and breakdown high protein foods etc - feeding primarily on flesh, bones and blood e.g. big cats, buzzards, crocodiles, hyenas.
- *Herbivores:* with teeth that are appropriate for cropping and chewing primarily on grass or other vegetation, with long digestive tracts (some with two stomachs) – examples of herbivores include deer, cattle, elephants, bison, rabbits, horses.
- *Graminivores:* all relatively small in size, feeding primarily on small food parcels such as grains and seeds, e.g. many birds and rodents.
- *Omnivores:* appropriate teeth for a mixed diet, feeding on a mixed diet of plants, roots and flesh, e.g. pigs, bears, badgers, the dog family, etc.
- *Frugivores:* feeding primarily (but not exclusively) on fruit and vegetation e.g. all primates such as lemurs, various monkeys, baboons, and the four species of 'anthropoid apes' – gorillas, chimpanzees and bonobos (our nearest genetic relatives, and *the most intelligent of the non-human great apes*), as well as orangutans and gibbons. Fruit eating bats which are *the most intelligent of bats* – and fruit eating parrots, which are *the most intelligent and long lived of all bird species*. Note: three very different branches of the whole evolutionary tree evolved their most intelligent species on specialized mainly fruit diets. Hmmmm?

The fundamental point here, in terms of **working with nature**, is to understand that due to its physiology/anatomy *every single creature on the planet gets everything it needs to be completely healthy if it eats its natural diet.* So if we determine our natural diet then we will know what foods will create and maintain natural health for us. *It is that simple.*

For solid evidence to help us be sure what our natural diet is, if you look at the size and shape of your guts, teeth, fingers, eyes and the nature of your digestive juices and saliva, and so on – all given to you by nature / evolution for a reason - you find that *your* 'canine teeth' or incisors (*and those of your ancient human ancestors*) are far smaller than those of chimpanzees and all other primates. This indicates that even amongst higher primates we are, and our ancestors were, the *least* adapted for killing and eating meat. Your canine teeth are, and those of early humans were, relatively useless as far as meat eating is concerned. Equally important, you *don't* have the big hard-wearing molars that are needed to grind up a diet of grass, tough leaves or grains.

However, you *do* have long intestines and low-acidity digestive juices – which are <u>*not*</u> suited to eating and processing meat or grains. And you do *not* have claws. Instead you have delicate

---

[33] Dennis Nelson, *Maximizing Your Nutrition*, First Printing (1988).

fingers, suited to delicate picking and peeling – and a relatively massive brain compared to body weight, and very sophisticated digestive system that can get enough energy out of a couple of ripe bananas for you to be able to cycle for a couple of hours. Looking beyond the body, you certainly won't find any fossilised cookers, deep-fryers or microwaves in our ancient human habitats!

So, anatomically the evidence points towards your human body having evolved by eating a raw diet, primarily made up of fruit, soft leaves and some nuts, roots and seeds - and probably some insects and eggs. Physiologically we can get everything that we need for health from our natural diet. However, if we eat an unnatural diet of processed grains and cooked fats/meats – (which we cook so they are safe or digestible, and precisely because *we are not designed to eat them* as primary foods) – then our health becomes a lottery, because our body cannot gain all it needs from them.[34]

Most people know and accept that the healthiest and healing foods are fruit and other raw foods – that's what we bring in to hospitals for sick friends and relatives. But to live on that really healthy raw fruit and veg alone?

Fruit was designed by nature to be attractive to eat so that fruiting plants could spread their seeds, using animals and birds to ensure their dispersal and ongoing survival. No other 'food' is designed by nature to be eaten in such a cooperative exchange, simple to digest and packed with the rewards for fruit eaters of a fantastic range of nutrients, delicious sweetness and wonderful flavours. So fruit eaters have a lovely and enjoyable time, and spread the seed, delivered to the earth with accompanying fertilizer. This is all about working with nature.

Are you getting how simple this 'working with nature' principle really is?

In peeling off hundreds of years of social, psychological and physiological conditioning as well as my own preconceptions, my research and experience of the issues suggests that eating and growing for an 'eat more raw' diet definitely *works with nature*, more than any other way of life. In temperate climates we are clearly not able to grow a tropical fruit diet for ourselves. However, with knowledge of organic horticulture, agroforestry and permaculture, alongside a science of natural and optimal nutrition, we can grow a huge and delicious variety of fruits, leaves, nuts and vegetables in ways that bring us close to a natural, optimal diet within this culture, whilst also creating personal and ecological health, working with nature as we go.

EVERYTHING GARDENS (OR EVERYTHING HAS EFFECTS)

This principle states that all parts of a system and inputs to that system affect its nature and how it operates and balances itself as a whole. Inputs or actions can have effects that are either positive or negative, or they can be more or less neutral. Permaculture seeks to consciously *work with inputs and relationships that create positive effects* - and to avoid inputs and relationships that create negative effects, working with neutral effects where that is useful.

---

[34] Chapters 2 & 3 in Tony Wright and Graham Gynn's book *Return to the Brain of Eden* (Inner Traditions, 2014) explain these issues far better and in far more detail – see the website http://leftinthedark.org.uk

All foods have some kind of positive or negative influence on us - they all 'garden' within our mind-body-spirit system. At this point, remember that at the Institute of Clinical Chemistry in Lausanne in the 1930s, Paul Kouchakoff demonstrated that the body's natural response to cooked foods is to treat them as foreign (i.e. unnatural) matter. This response, called 'digestive leucocytosis', involves the immune system sending a rush of white blood cells – leucocytes – to the intestines to deal with the foreign matter. This occupies the immune system and reduces its capacity makes to fight other bodily invaders. This does not happen with raw foods. It also does not occur when something raw is eaten immediately before starting to eat something cooked.[35]

A simple explanation to this is that cooking changes the chemical composition of foods. Raw foods are built of 'natural' chemicals, created by nature, so the body has an innate ability to recognise them as natural. Cooked foods, particularly highly processed foods, contain numerous 'de-natured' chemical compounds, as the heating and processing changes the structure of natural chemicals. Therefore the body cannot recognise them and reacts to them as foreign matter, creating the immune response described above. Some of these chemical concoctions it throws out straight away. Many others it can't recognize or deal with so they are stored in the body – particularly in the fats – and they gradually have a degenerating effect because they don't have a useful, natural role. However, just by being there they have an effect. They clog up the body's systems, influence the growth of cells in an unnatural way or have other adverse effects.

Natural, health creating foods give cells what they need, which is a vibrant body that can efficiently digest and assimilate nutrients and reproduce healthy cells. So this principle implies eating ecologically sound foods with *health creating effects* - and avoiding foods with negative effects. This is applied common sense. Many cooked and inorganic foods act like agrochemicals, doing a job, with their damaging long term effects well hidden. You can't see the agrochemicals in non-organic food or in the soil. Equally you can't see the toxins in fried and processed foods. They are both well hidden, but have unavoidable and eventually visible long term effects.

In the economic 'garden', there are the effects of where and how you spend your money. Like watering or feeding a plant, our spending always feeds some economic entity, spreading through a mycorrhisal web to its suppliers, employees, managers, owners and so on. Buying local and organic, you feed a positive chain in the economy. And if you buy elsewhere then you may feed harmful effects within the environmental and socio-economic ecosystems. So spend 'your' money and energy consciously and positively. *The same goes for your contribution to the world through work – which is normally your biggest economic impact.* Remember that.

My experience is that an 'eat more raw' lifestyle, with balanced use of different types of fruit and raw foods can be used to promote natural health and tackle illness, at a personal and planetary level. Organic growing, forest gardening, permaculture and agroforestry create positive effects, inside and out, through their web of effects. Toxic foods create and maintain a toxic environment in our bodies and beyond, whilst healthy foods create a healthy environment in our bodies and beyond. It's all gardening really!

---

[35] See digestive leucocytosis in Susannah & Leslie Kenton's *The New Raw Energy*, Vermillion (1994), p.41 & 89.

MAXIMUM OUTPUT FOR MINIMUM EFFORT

This principle is about maximizing beneficial effects by making minimal but carefully thought-through changes – sometimes described as 'make small changes for big effects'.

By eating health-creating foods, improved health is achieved with relatively little effort. These foods also generally: a) need less work to prepare and clean up after; b) use significantly less packaging and containers; c) use much less energy than in cooking and storing; and d) do not reduce or destroy the food value of vitamins, enzymes and minerals.

Maximum output, minimum effort is also achieved because:
- Undamaged vitamins, minerals *and* enzymes work together as a nutritional 'guild', where each element benefits the other, working together so that their whole effect is definitely greater than the sum of their constituent parts.[36]
- We need undamaged essential amino acids and EFAs (Essential Fatty Acids) to be strong and healthy.[37] Cooking kills the enzymes in food that are vital for assimilation of amino acids and EFAs, as most food enzymes are destroyed above about 42°c. A balanced and varied raw food diet provides all the essential amino acids and EFAs.
- Ripe fruit tastes delicious, taking about half an hour to digest on an empty stomach.[38]

Meanwhile very many cooked and processed foods and meals take many hours and lots of work to digest, particularly when different food types are combined. Cooking requires work to process and prepare, careful storing to keep it 'safe' and lots of clearing up. So cooked food usually = more input + less output. And great pleasure often arises when you *eat more raw* because your body enjoys what it is naturally designed to eat. It can take time to adjust and learn what you like best, but *nature and evolution definitely designed pleasure into the equation*. If you go to some raw food preparation classes and use Part 10 of this book, that'll be a fast-track MOME (Max-Output-Min-Effort) approach to learning some really delicious recipes.

Via the food chain, ultimately all animal protein is built from the plant based amino acids that are the building blocks of life because that is *the most efficient way nature has created to build protein in larger animals*. So it's *maximum output for minimum effort*, in terms of land, energy use, pollution, protein building and so on, when we obtain our amino acids direct from good plant sources rather from animal protein (see *The Protein Question* a few pages further on).

A well-designed diet with roughly 50%+ raw foods can create many positive 'ripple effects', with big benefits achieved through relatively smaller changes – for example:
- *Physical, Mental and Spiritual Health Benefits*: a well-designed natural diet promotes health and vitality on all levels, in the short and long term
- *Ecological Benefits*: reduces energy use, waste, packaging, water and land demand; promotes landscape, wildlife and biodiversity, and generally means more tree crops

---

[36] 'Guilds' are defined and described in more detail in the useful plants section (p.143).

[37] For essential amino acids lists & food sources for them see raw food books in Appendices, Wikipedia, etc.

[38] Ripeness it is the state fruit is meant to be eaten in. Supermarkets are *not* good if you want to know what ripe fruit tastes and feels like, as unripe fruit allows for easier handling and storage for them.

- *Compassionate Benefits*: reduces human suffering by promoting health, rather than creating illness, and avoids animal suffering
- *Economic Benefits*: promotes positively directed spending; can cut food costs, e.g if you get into food growing, permaculture and indoor sprouting; can cut energy costs; can massively reduce health-care costs, and avoid supporting economic exploitation within the unsustainable global food production industry.[39] Healthier nutrition will significantly reduce the huge long term health care costs that society will *have to* pay for (i.e. you the payer of tax, health insurance, treatment, etc). Invest in health creation, don't just pay up for insurance against the costs of illness!

Some of the typical effects, which create big benefits when added together, are:
- Feeling more vital and alive, with more energy – the single most common benefit that people most widely *feel* and experience from eating more raw.
- Improved senses of taste and smell, generally more sensitivity, so food tastes great.
- Clearer head and more awake.
- Clear, healthy skin, with little or no B.O. (except during a 'detox') - a sweet smelling body in fact - reduced need for soaps, shampoos and less smelly clothes;
- A better and more positive understanding of one's body and one's bodily functions;
- Far less packaging or waste - no food tins, aluminium cans, frozen food packs, etc.
- Less kitchen clutter – fewer jars, bottles of sauce, food tins, packets, saucepans, etc.
- Less use of energy: no need for a freezer, and ultimately no need for a fridge or cooker if you choose to go all the way.

Eating more raw foods can also be an easy, healthy way to lose a few unhealthy pounds (weight that is!). Angela Stokes is a particularly inspiring example of using a much improved diet to lose a lot of weight – in Angela's case from 297lb/127kg (over 21 stone) to less than half that weight at 138lb/62kg (under ten stone) – 'half the weight, twice the life' as she puts it!![40] You can eat as much delicious raw foods as you want and if you are over-weight you will still lose pounds, and feel much better as a result.

Anyone who's particularly interested in fitness should read Dr Doug Graham's books or website (see Appendix 3) to learn about the superior health, fitness and strength that is achievable with a raw food lifestyle. Alternatively, Mike Nash's book *Aggressive Health* and Stephen Arlin's book *Raw Power* cover super-fitness and strength training from a raw perspective – all achieving results with different types of raw diet. So all over the world there are very many raw foodists who are very fit men and women who run, walk, cycle, dance, do lots of yoga and so on. There's quite a few raw yogini's these days in fact.

So, in numerous ways an 'eat more raw' diet maximises positive effects with minimum effort, creating many significant positive effects through carefully thought-out changes.

---

[39] *The Food System*, by Tansey and Worsley (Earthscan, 1995), is an excellent book on the global food industry, and a 30 minute online talk by Geoff Tansey at http://www.tansey.org.uk/news/FStalk.html

[40] See Angela's excellent website and Raw Reform e-books at www.rawreform.com

YIELD IS (THEORETICALLY) UNLIMITED

In theory changes can always be made to a system to increase its yield. So a house can be built just to be a dwelling – or can also be built to save energy ... and to generate energy ... to be educational ... be beautiful and spiritually inspiring ... and to generate income, for example by having space to run courses. This indicates how to raise the yield of a house.

More research and experience will help clarify the multiple benefits (or yields) of an eat more raw lifestyle, and will depend on the application of high quality information and knowledge in a range of relevant situations. The greatest long term benefits will arise as one generation passes a more complete culture of health to the next. The critical stages are to pass on health at conception, and during pregnancy and infancy. Whilst extensive research has confirmed that breastfeeding raises IQ, an early years diet of only human breast milk and fruit/raw foods will not automatically create happy, brilliant people – raising children is clearly far more complicated than that, with parental imprinting, Continuum Concept factors and other influences being highly important.[41] However, on average, breastfeeding and a positive diet can help very significantly, giving a child a better start, and having an influence through the rest of life. Breastfeeding is almost certainly the single most important thing because nature designed breast milk to be the ideal food for babies, plus this creates a sense of security which has numerous benefits and yields over a lifetime. Furthermore there is a clear relationship in the animal and cetacean world between extended breast-feeding and large brain size. There is also an increasing clear body of evidence to suggest that extended breastfeeding beyond 1 year old has significant benefits which are greater than if breastfeeding is limited to 1 year or less.[42]

Optimum nutrition will inevitably provide an excellent start for children and yield many benefits through life. Combined with living in sustainable, beautiful and supportive communities and neighbourhoods, the potential benefits and 'yield' may be enormous - both in the present and the future - as more people explore what it means in practice. In adults who adjust to a well designed eat more raw lifestyle the benefits and yields will depend on the individual and the diet chosen – yields are likely to include improved health, more energy, better mental clarity, higher self-esteem and improved self-image, more motivated, reduced fear of illness, reduced negative environmental and economic impacts, and so on. Designing in more yields can be part of the fun of making the transition.

THE PROBLEM IS THE SOLUTION

Along with *working with nature* this is perhaps the most powerful attitude principle to instill in yourself. The profound wisdom, and great simplicity of this principle is that real solutions arise from understanding and responding to the deeper nature of the problem.

A poor diet is linked to great human suffering, for those that become sick themselves and for family and friends as a result of the illness. In wealthy nations this suffering often arises from

---

[41] See Jean Liedloff, *The Continuum Concept*, De Capo Press (1986) – an important book; also see *The Mother* magazine (published by Art of Change).

[42] See Veronica Robinson's book *The Drinks Are On Me*, Art of Change (2007).

avoidable lifestyle / diet-related chronic illness e.g. heart disease, cancer and diabetes. In poorer nations this suffering is often caused by a lack of food, key nutrients and dietary diversity – often worsened by wealthy nations and global institutions imposing inappropriate western agricultural practices and trading conditions upon poorer nations, as conditions for loans (i.e. debt) and 'aid', and by western companies selling wholly inappropriate foods to the innocent – such as Nestlé's sales of artificial milk to nursing mothers in Africa, despite concerted public protests.[43]

We've said it before but we'll say it again - many of the wealthier nations are amongst the sickest in the world, on many levels:

- Americans consume more food per head than any other nation – they are the most obese and have the highest incidence of calcium deficiency. 70% of Americans over 40 suffer from at least one degenerative disease.
- Australians eat more red meat per head than any other nation – they also have the highest incidence of cancer.
- Scotland has one of the worst records of diet related chronic illness[44] - and UK adult obesity rates have almost quadrupled in the last 25 years, with 24.9% of people obese and the UK topping the obesity league in western Europe (source: NHS Choices).

The wealthier nations also have the highest carbon emissions per head and resource use per head. So levels of chronic ill-health and chronic *un*sustainability are both clearly 'significant problems' for our wealthy societies - and as Albert Einstein said:

We cannot solve the significant problems of our time at the same level of thinking that created them; we have to move to a new level of thinking.

In terms of diet, nutrition and health, how do we move to 'a new level of thinking'? And more specifically what does it mean in practice? Does it mean just moving to a new school of ideas or opinions? Or does it mean *a deeper level of understanding and response to the deeper nature of the significant problems* to create the significant solutions?

A new level of thinking means: *a) an attitude and approach that actively seeks to understand and <u>create</u> real health <u>at all levels</u>, in all areas of life; and b) finding ways of doing things where health and sustainability arise <u>naturally</u> from our actions, behaviours and ways of thinking.*

This needs an entirely different way of perceiving food and its relationship to health, so that food and its production become *tools with which we create health* - social, economic and environmental health – at the same time as food being something to enjoy and sustain us naturally. And it means food being one critical component to health, but not the only one.[45]

The western agro-industrial, meat'n'wheat culture is used and abused by corporations that forcefully spread it around the world, creating farming dependence on single crops, genetically

---

[43] For more information contact Baby Milk Action - www.babymilkaction.org

[44] Sources: *Sustainable Somerset New Digest 28*; Permaculture Introductory Course with Phil Corbett, Leicester, Spring 1994; Dr Joel Robbins CD, *Health Through Nutrition* (Health & Wellness Center).

[45] Dr Joel Robbins *Attitudes to Health* CDs (Health & Wellness Center) address several of these issues.

manipulated seeds, and costly pesticides and fertilisers supplied by multi-nationals. This destroys the self-reliance of developing countries, both agricultural and economic, and consciously creates impoverishment, debt and dependency in order to sustain the global growth of trade and the economic dominance of a small minority of corporations.

There are other, much more loving ways to treat people and planet, which are more efficient and effective in meeting human needs (e.g. agroforestry systems). The traditional western diet or what's known as SAD (Standard American Diet) involves a great deal of wasteful energy use and pollution, whilst it also actively damages both human and ecological health – particularly in the long term. So a 'normal' diet and 'normal' agriculture are a very clear 'lose: lose' multiple problem creating situation. Meanwhile, an organic 50%+ raw diet seems much more like a 'win: win' multi-solution creating situation.

In practice, the current western diet, and industrialised food production, marketing and trading systems are clearly linked to a vast range of physical and psychological health problems; to exploitative economic systems and environmental destruction; and to considerable animal suffering. So food and agriculture are central to health and sustainability problems. Changing our understanding, our thinking, our attitudes and our activities in these areas is *the* solution. Well-designed positive changes in all these 4 areas – understanding, thinking, attitudes and activities - *will* improve the quality of economic development, improve our quality of life, increase our sustainability and raise individual and social levels of health. So how about designing your diet and lifestyle to be consciously part of the solution, at all levels?

The simplest and most direct problem-solution response is a) to change what you eat, b) change how you obtain your food, and c) change who and where you get it from.

HARVEST ONLY SUNSHINE (OR CLOSING THE LOOP)

Ultimately all life energy on earth is derived from the sun's energy. What's more there is no such thing as waste in nature. Think about this for a moment, because it's absolutely true, and it contains the essence of nature's absolute and fundamental efficiency.

So 'Closing the loop' means designing our lives, diets and living systems so that all energy and resources are cycled back into nature, food production and remanufacturing with nothing wasted. A locally and organically produced eat more raw lifestyle is a simple way to get closer to sustainable energy and resource use and closed loop systems in our eating and food production. The simpler your diet the less energy you use and the simpler it is to re-cycle your food waste. The more natural and less processed your food is then the easier it is to compost, and the more quickly it can return to the nutrient cycle.

The sun's energy combines with the energy of life to give us everything we need – vitamins, minerals, enzymes, amino-acids, carbohydrates, EFAs and water – in the best form, and the ideal form. Fruit is sunlight turned into sugars and vitamins in particular. Green leaves are sunlight turned into chlorophyll, amino acids and minerals in particular. Eating them fresh and raw is the most direct way to harvest only sunshine. Positive approaches to creating health, improve vitality, self-reliance, creativity, positive thinking and quality of life, and also create aharvest of smiling faces: human sunshine.

We all have choices about the cause-and-effect food chain that we sit hungrily at the end of. So which do you choose? Problem causing food chains, or solution causing food chains?

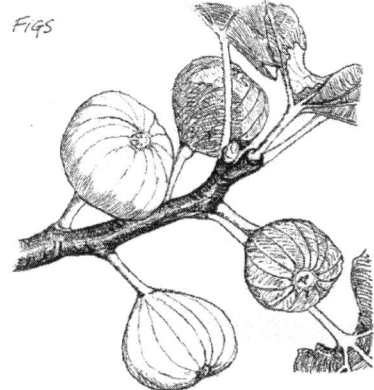

A highly sustainable, roughly 50%+ raw diet works with nature because it is rooted in an understanding of life's natural processes of health creation and our basic natural needs. What is more, it provides the opportunity for numerous improved yields, it creates lots of positive effects within us and beyond us, it creates numerous solutions to numerous problems, it harvests sunshine very directly and closes many loops, and also creates many big and positive effects from making relatively small changes in our lives.

The problem IS the solution, and working with nature IS the natural way to vibrant health. Imagine the health impacts when at least 5% to 10% of the population is eating at least 50% raw, supplied by sustainable food growing systems. Think of the knock-on effects for the health service, in agriculture and the food supply industry. Sit for a few minutes, and imagine this as a possible future and imagine your place in it... We could just be at the tipping point for a peaceful and positive, healthy revolution ... starting in some of our lives, in some communities and in some social networks.

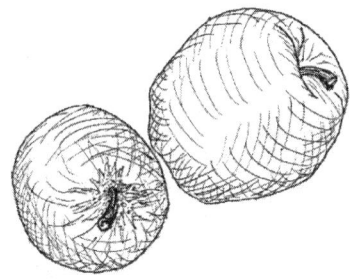

For an interpretation of the eat more raw lifestyle within the *Holmgren Principles* of permaculture, see the *eat more raw* website.

SOME 'FREQUENTLY ASKED QUESTIONS' ABOUT RAW FOODS

THE COOKING QUESTION

The first question is "so what's so bad about cooking? Everyone's does it!"

The answer to this question is to say that cooking happens for understandable reasons – it's not saying cooking is wrong. The issue is what is cooked, how it's cooked and why. It's about considering cooking and its relationship to nature and a) health as a state, and b) the creation of health as a process. It's about developing a sense of what optimum nutrition is, an optimum diet, and the short and long term healthy survival, development and success of the human species - for our body and organs, brain and neurological system, and for our reproductive systems and the growth of each new generation. That's what it's about.

On one level it's simply about the different kinds of biochemistry of different kinds of foods, and *the hidden effects* of these chemical differences. On another level it's about understanding the *molecular effects* of different levels of heat. Temperature is in effect a measure of the speed and degree of movement of molecules. At the molecular level heating will cause the breakdown of a form of molecular stability within living things that, in the vast majority of living things, occurs within a very narrow temperature band from around zero degrees to around forty degrees centigrade. Most life cannot survive outside that band. So what we call 'cooking' changes the molecular structure – it makes many inedible things edible, and many things that are dangerous to eat (e.g. because of parasites, etc) relatively less dangerous. At the same time, on the level of sophisticated molecular engineering it renders our building blocks and fuels crude and lifeless. Raising heat levels denatures proteins at around 55-65 degrees C. It also dissolves many vital minerals out of foods (e.g. vegetables) into the water they are cooked in.

Cooking happens, will continue to happen around us, and has a major role in almost all cultures. However, we are higher primates in physiological, biological and anatomical terms. And we can never get away from that basic fact. Since mankind's emergence in the equatorial forests we have spread to harsher northern climates where we have relied on foods that we did not evolve to eat and which are not good if eaten raw by humans. Northern ecosystems have massively less plant diversity, with less than 40 native tree species in Britain, compared to around 6000 in tropical forests i.e. 150 times more diverse than Britain. Therefore there are far fewer naturally digestible plant foods because of that reduced diversity - and because there is less of the sun's energy to grow and ripen things.[46] So to survive in this environment we had to cook to make things sufficiently edible and turn them into 'food'. So cooking is not 'wrong'.

The cooking question is about looking at where we are now, understanding the health and ecological effects of our food habits, and choosing where we want to be in the present and future. The state of western culture shows clearly that *we cannot and will not reach health, in this generation or in future generations if we continue with the current western diet and the agro-industrial food system that goes hand in hand with it.*

---

[46] Colin Tudge's book, *The Secret Life of Trees*, Penguin (2006) is a wonderful source of information about every aspects of trees and their vital role in life as a whole on this planet.

Put simply, it doesn't take a genius to see that *between three to ten generations of the typical modern western diet would be nothing less than a disaster for the human species* – in social, health, economic, reproductive and evolutionary terms.

Nature doesn't cook her foods for any creature; not one - it is not part of any natural systems of life or ecology. And she certainly doesn't super-process them. So this question is about *researching and discovering what optimum nutrition is for us humans in the current age*, taking into account what is practical and realistic, and what is inspiring and challenging yet possible. And about using permaculture to create food-growing systems that meet the needs of that optimum diet. *A well-designed, nutrient rich and alkaline roughly 50%+ raw diet is a practical and realistic initial target to aim for* - some may take time and need support to achieve it - many others can achieve it in a relatively quickly and easily. That leaves up to 50% for cooking, and if that is your choice then whole foods and alkalinity are key to health.

Despite what I thought a few years ago I now know *from experience* that I do not need to cook food to live and thrive. I know *from experience* that I am both happier and healthier on a diet with little or no cooked foods, and that it feels really good. So I'm not suggesting you have to give up cooking – have a go at the 50% raw target for at least 28 days and then see how it feels.

THE PROTEIN QUESTION

"So where do you get your protein from then?"

Look at the strength of any gorilla that happens to stroll by and ask where it gets its protein! Gorillas are the strongest primates. They normally eat mainly leaves and shoots, and a little fruit (because of availability rather than choice) – and they're very laid back too! As are our closest genetic relatives, Bonobos. Either could probably rip your arm off, although they're not likely to. So where do they get their strength from? Great apes thrive on a low protein diet. Yet they are incredibly strong, because they get all the amino-acids they need to *build* protein and muscle from a fruit and leaf based diet. Equally, all the super-strong 'beasts of burden' are herbivores.

> *We build or replace our muscles and other tissues by assembling the component parts, the amino acids and proteins, into fresh protein according to the plan of our DNA. To use protein from beef directly to make our muscles would be like taking the parts of a tractor to repair a washing machine.* James Lovelock, The Revenge of Gaia, p.23

So how much protein do humans actually need? Can nature give us any clues? Well, human breast milk has no more than 2% to 3% protein, which is very low in comparison with many other animals, and that's at the time in life when we need more protein to build our growing baby bodies. Human breast milk is a perfectly designed natural food – a rich and nutrient dense diet. It tells us a lot about our protein needs. What we need are the building blocks that enable our body to build its own proteins. So in fact the protein question is a very interesting and important one. What is emerging is that there actually appear to be significant negative factors associated with a high protein diet – and such a diet tends to go hand in hand with a high cooked and processed animal fat diet. There are two particular protein-disease relationships of interest: protein and osteoporosis, and protein and cancer.

The growth of osteoporosis, especially amongst users of concentrated protein such as athletes and body builders, now suggests that a high protein diet is positively unhealthy. A high protein diet creates acidity as more acidic digestive juices are needed to break down protein. A carnivore's digestive juices are about 10 times more acid than ours, so they break meat down quickly and get it out fast (and kill accompanying bacteria and parasites), before it putrefies badly.

A high-protein-eating, acid-creating human body is normally not getting the minerals it needs in a normal cooked and processed diet. So the only place it can get minerals from are its own mineral stores – particularly our bones – which it therefore has to use to balance the body's pH and the blood's pH, because if the blood goes out of a very narrow neutral to slightly alkaline range we die. So survival over-rides health again. In this way the depletion of calcium in the bones (osteoporosis) is linked to a demineralised diet, because other minerals and vitamins, and not only calcium, are needed for healthy bones because they are catalysts required in the bone building process. Remember, osteoporosis is considered 'normal' for older Americans these days - or we should say, osteoporosis is considered normal for anyone who has eaten a typical American diet for a lengthy period, whether in the US, Britain or anywhere.

The China Study by T Colin Campbell PhD details the results of 'the most comprehensive study of nutrition ever conducted', with eminent US and UK universities involved, covering 65 countries, 130 villages and 6,500 adults and their families. It sets out the results of detailed long term research which show a very *clear correlation between cooked animal protein and various forms of cancer*, with aflotoxin having an apparently significant role as a cancer promoter. Low animal protein countries / diets were seen to have a significantly lower incidence of cancer.

So, essential amino-acids (not primary protein) are critical for us to receive in our diet as they allow the body to build proteins itself, and therefore to build and maintain our muscles according to our own DNA code, which determines what our body needs. This is why in nutrition there is a category of nutrients called *essential amino acids*, and there is *not* a category called essential proteins. We can easily obtain all the essential protein building amino-acids we need from vegetables, seeds, nuts and even fruit – green leafy vegetables being the real wonders. If you want to look into this question more you'll find the answers in Dr Doug Graham's books, *The Sunfood Diet Success System* by David Wolfe and *The China Study* by T Colin Campbell PhD.

THE FAT QUESTION

Turning to the fat question, the key thing is that vegetable fats in their natural, unprocessed and uncooked state are essentially 'good', within limits, whilst processed and cooked fats (vegetable or animal) are essentially 'bad', because heating and processing fats and oils corrupts their structure, particularly when heated to high temperatures. This is significant because fats in our bodies are our hormone factories and our hormones are 'switches' that determine how our genes are read. So putting corrupted fats into our body creates corrupted outcomes.

Our organs and glands are significantly built from fats. So, when a typical diet contains many corrupted fats and proteins, cancers appear in our organs and glands, as cancers are corruptions of the cell regeneration process. So it is almost inevitable that cancers will emerge through a lifetime of consuming corrupted fats and corrupted proteins – so any idea that we can 'cure cancer' without changing our diet and lifestyle reflects very weird view of nature.

Dr Udo Erasmus' excellent book or tape *Fats That Heal, Fats That Kill* is a fantastic source of information for understanding the dangers of the bad fats, such as those in so many margarines and cooking oils – as well as the healing power of good fats.[47]

Also, processed foods are not whole foods, so where processed foods include processed fats, the fats have been separated from all or some of the fibre, vitamins and so on, which they are combined with in their natural state and which help them to be assimilated if eaten in their natural state. Processing of any form involves extra energy use, packaging and transport, and is often just another case of someone pushing a new processed food to keep their profits up.

There are various opinions amongst raw food advocates on the issue of 'healthy' raw fats from plant sources. Dr Douglas Graham and Fred Paténaude are amongst those who believe that controlling our fat intake is very important, even if it is high quality and raw. Doug Graham points out that the standard American diet (SAD) obtains 42% of its calories from its fat intake, and this is similar for vegans and vegetarians – for some raw fooders it's just as high. Meanwhile, I have heard David Wolfe joke that 'you can never eat too many avocados'[48], whilst also advocating pure raw coconut oil as a fabulous food. Part of Dave Wolfe's argument is that good quality fats are needed *to dissolve the bad fats which are stored in our body*, because water (including the water in fruits/veg) cannot dissolve or break down fats (which is why soaps are made from fat/oil). Wolfe also always emphasizes the importance of green leafy vegetables, and only promotes raw fats within the context of a balanced raw vegan diet.

More recently Tony Wright has emphasized the critical role of high quality raw plant-based fats in neurological development and maintenance, particularly for pregnant and nursing mothers, toddlers and children.[49] Wright's biochemical logic suggests that our natural, 'evolutionary' diet would be very likely have included a higher proportion of *high quality fats* and minerals than our closest genetic relatives (bonobos and chimpanzees) because we have a bigger brain, which is basically a large lump of amazingly complex fatty tissue and crystalline minerals, for which vegetable fatty acids are the ideal building and maintenance materials.

Meanwhile Doug Graham, whose expertise is in athletic performance, states that fats, whether cooked or raw, clog up the cardiovascular system, and reduce the oxygen carrying capacity of the blood. He says that to deal with excessive fats the body releases more adrenaline, and the pancreas produces higher levels of insulin for the body to deal with the fats in the bloodstream. Dr Graham cites the recommendations of the Pritkin Longevity Center, which he says has 'the finest health-regeneration record of any organisation in the US'. They recommend no more than 10% fat in your diet, and using this as a base Doug Graham states that 80/10/10 is the optimum health target – 80% of calories from simple carbohydrates (from fruit sugars), with 10% fat and 10% protein.

---

[47] See http://www.udoerasmus.com/fatsmain.htm

[48] This was probably in the mid-late 1990's, so whether David Wolfe still says this I do not know, although I understand that he still emphasises the vital role of high quality fats in the diet for various reasons.

[49] Visit http://www.kaleidos.org.uk/home.htm#OVERVIEW, and scroll down to Chapter 2: Construction Materials, or see the book *Return to the Brain of Eden*, by Tony Wright and Graham Gynn.

Certainly Doug Graham and the professional athletes he advises are evidence in themselves that you can enjoy an extremely high level of fitness on a low fat, low protein, high fruit, raw diet. Equally however, the sharp minds and information storage capacity of Wolfe (who's also very fit) and Wright also indicate that a higher percentage of highest quality fats can also produce good results. Dr Udo Erasmus's website also stresses another perspective:

Healing fats are required, together with other nutrients, to prevent and reverse so-called "incurable" degenerative diseases: heart disease, cancer, and Type II diabetes. Healing fats also help reverse arthritis, obesity, PMS, allergies, asthma, skin conditions, fatigue, yeast and fungal infections, addictions, certain types of mental illness, and many other conditions.

So the points of difference within the raw movement are what the best balance is - all agree that the inclusion of high quality raw fats (10% minimum) from plant sources is vitally important.

In warm weather and warm climates I have felt great eating a small amount of raw vegetable fats in my diet (from avocados, oils, nuts and / or seeds). I've also felt good eating higher proportions of fats in cooler climates, although never great if I eat above about 20%. So I've found climate is a factor in dietary fat. My sense is that 10%-20% of calories from high quality fats can produce excellent results depending on age, climate and the balance of the rest the diet, levels of exercise, attitude, dietary history, current health and, importantly, what you may be wanting or needing to shift out of the body in terms of pollutants and toxins.

It's vital to get out of the simplistic 'fats are bad' mindset. The right kinds of raw, unprocessed fats are not only good, they are *essential* – and more so in a cleansing phase to break down and shift the bad fats out, as well as during pregnancy and breast feeding, and for infants and children – to build healthy brains and organs – 10% would probably be too little.

The key is to find the level that suits you within reason, and to include the best quality fats in your diet. Examples of foods with these good quality fats are: raw cold pressed and refrigerated flax and hemp oil, Udo's Choice oil blend; raw flax, pumpkin, sunflower, sesame and hemp seeds; raw coconut oil/butter, raw cacao butter, and algae oil / DHA supplements; raw fatty fruits such as avocado and durian, and fresh coconut. And of course many of these high quality fat foods also contain numerous vitamins and minerals (as well as protein).

THE MEAT QUESTION

"So what about chimpanzees eating meat then?"

Yes, chimps have been found to eat meat and we humans can and do eat meat of course. Does this mean it is best for our mind-body system and the planetary system to do so? We can do many things and survive or enjoy them, but that does not mean they good for us. Looking at it a different way, do you prefer the smell of a fruit 'n' veg warehouse or a slaughter house?

All I can say is that I feel better in my mind, body and spirit not eating meat. I am not into meat-eater bashing. For much of my life I was a meat eater, until my mid-twenties (about 1987). This was linked to my walks in the beautiful Hampshire countryside where I found well hidden battery chicken houses with a grey atmosphere of death and disease; saw lorries passing through Alton and Petersfield town centres crammed with thousands of boxed-in chickens on their way to the slaughterhouse; and was not able to find a chicken in the supermarket with a straight spine or unbroken legs - I started to make the links. My changes from being a meat eater have combined logic based on sound information from people and sources that I trust, alongside a strong sense of what feels right for me and what I want to do.

As for the common retort 'but chimpanzees eat meat', let's get stuck into that and explore it properly. Yes, some chimpanzees do eat meat – they eat meat from time to time, not everyday, and not several times a day, and not cooked – it's always raw. The behaviour associated with a chimpanzee's meat eating is important to note – it often involves a frenzied and barbaric slaughter of monkeys. The leading primate researcher, Jane Goodall, also found that it was sometimes even cannibalistic and apparently psychopathic.

Humans have a very different moral, ethical and contemplative capacity to chimpanzees. We can consider and digest more information, both rational and ethical, and in doing so we make decisions. Some humans kill people; it doesn't mean I should. The Olympic athletes of ancient Greece were fed mainly fruit; their soldiers on the other hand were fed meat.

Suggesting that we should eat meat because chimpanzees have been found to eat meat is to me a rather bizarre form of logic. But if this logic is used then the essentially fruitarian habits of orangutans and bonobos, and the mainly leaf-eating habits of gorillas are equally relevant. So, let's follow it through, and look at a number of relevant issues logically:

1. We have much smaller canine teeth than chimps, which logically suggests we are *less* suited to meat eating than chimpanzees.
2. The chimpanzee logic implies we should *always* eat our meat fresh and raw, and should kill it ourselves – by hand.
3. It also suggests that *the vast bulk of what we eat should be fresh, ripe, raw fruit and leaves as chimpanzees do* - with some flowers and honey, as well as nice juicy insects and grubs, and only a small amount of raw meat. How do you fancy that?
4. Finally the logic suggests we should pay closer attention to our closest genetic/DNA relative, the Bonobo, which a) are more placid and more intelligent than their heavier relatives, b) eat mainly fruit, as well as leaves, flowers, bark, stems, roots, insect larvae, worms, crustaceans, honey, eggs, and soil and occasionally small animals c) lb for lb are much stronger than us. They live in close and affectionate groups, using sexual interaction rather than violence when they feel stress, and they also have a matriarchal society. Make of that what you will.[50]

So if you want to use the 'chimpanzees and meat' argument, the logic is clear and simple.

Another aspect of this is that the environmental costs of meat eating are massive. A key element of the very lengthy McLibel trial was the claimed association between Big Macs and rainforest destruction for short-term cattle ranching, which was not legally proven, although many sources show the vast devastation that is associated with large scale animal farming / meat production.[51] Simon Fairlie's book *Meat: A Benign Extravagance* makes good arguments about

---

[50] See http://www.animalfactguide.com/animal-facts/bonobo/

[51] For example, *Bringing The Food Economy Home*, Helena Norberg Hodge et al, Zed Books (2002).

the ecologically beneficial role that animal farming *can* make – however, *mainly* animal farming is an ecological disaster, that is a long way from being carried out in the ways Simon calls for, and will remain so for the foreseeable future so long as there are arguments to justify the majority of people wanting cheap and plentiful meat. Of course none of this addresses our pre-supposed 'right' to farm animals for the purpose of slaughtering them and eating them. So, yes, we are incredibly adaptable, and yes we can eat meat - but it is increasingly obvious that our high meat consumption is both a narrow socio-cultural norm and a physical and economic addiction that is generating significant costs in terms of human and environmental health.

THE STARCH AND CARBOHYDRATE QUESTION

"But what about starch and carbohydrates then?"

Along with fat and protein, carbohydrates are one of three dietary macronutrients that provide calories. It is generally understood that carbohydrates provide most of our bodies' energy needs, although at the cellular level ATP (adrinosine triphosphate) is the store and source of our energy - carbohydrates (starches and sugars), proteins and fats are converted into ATP.

The chemical structure of carbohydrates determines whether they are the 'simple' or 'complex' types. Both of these types contain four calories per gram and both are turned into glucose (the only sugar that our body uses), which is then used in the cellular ATP cycle. Simple carbohydrates are digested quickly and include fruits, fruit juice, milk, yoghurt, honey, molasses and sugar. Complex carbohydrates take longer to digest and typically include cooked starchy vegetables, breads, cereals, legumes and pasta. It's not as easy as saying one type is good and one is bad, as raw fruit sugars are a very different story to refined sugar. Also bananas, for example, contain both simple and complex carbohydrates, giving a balanced energy release over time. Starches have to be turned into glucose and this involves more work for the body in comparison with taking those sugars directly from fruit.

Again looking at our anatomy and physiology, and our digestive system, we are very clearly not graminivores designed by nature to eat grains (or grain products) – all grain eating mammals are small.[52] Highly processed starches clog up the digestive system a great deal, especially when combined with cooked fats. Conventional nutritionists now recommend that we should avoid refined sugars and that we should gain most of our simple carbohydrates from foods that also contain vitamins and minerals, such as fruits, milks or yoghurts.

So the point is, we do not need starch in our diet although we do need carbohydrates. Like the other two key macronutrients, it is quite possible to gain all the carbohydrates we need, both simple and complex, from raw fruits, vegetables, nuts, seeds and soaked or sprouted raw whole grains.

If we placed the emphasis on the obtaining a good supply of micronutrients from natural sources (vitamins, minerals, Essential Fatty Acids, food enzymes), rather than the macronutrients (proteins, carbs, fats), then we'd be a much healthier bunch.

---

[52] See Dr Douglas Graham's excellent booklet *Grain Damage* for more info on the subject of grains.

The Nutritional & Health Research Question

This is a really important question, because nutritional research and conventional nutritional science has played a central role in shaping our cultural understanding of food, and our idea about what is good or bad for us to eat, as well as what is normal to eat.

For most of us, our dietary choices are culturally determined by what we perceive as 'normal' and by what the food industry offers us. Most people's food choices are clearly *not* based on study, unbiased information or a cultural attitude that seeks to create and maintain vibrant health.

Having sat on many senior US food and nutrition committees, T Colin Campbell developed a very clear understanding of how the nutritional research system works in practice. His book *The China Study* makes very clear how the official view of nutrition has been shaped by the politically and economically powerful food and farming industry, and how food industry interests have suppressed research that indicates *the standard western diet is fundamentally unhealthy*. In *The China Study*, T Colin Campbell does a hugely important (and courageous) job of exposing the often corrupted or distorted nature of health research, nutritional science and health and diet advisory committees in the USA – I recommend it to anyone wanting to understand these issues.[53] For example, a long term study of thousands of people in the USA indicated that meat eaters were 2 to 3 times more likely to suffer from dementia than vegetarians – but despite its huge implications the researchers were unable to gain funding to take their studies further, and the research results were suppressed over time.

The problem with nutritional research is not that it comes up with 'wrong' answers, or that scientific technique is flawed. The problem is that it's starting point and questions are largely based on hidden assumptions and/or vested interests. Cooked foods and the standard western diet is the base line of what is 'normal' in our society and 'normal' for most nutrition researchers – and for the organisations that fund them. Nutritional research and nutritional science does not start with a clean sheet, and is often paid to ask the wrong questions. So many well paid 'food scientists' work on the development of highly processed, unhealthy foods – yet **there is no large established body of scientific research into health creation** - think hard about that fact.

In fact, there is more genuine, objective science in primate nutrition research in zoos than there is in the field of human nutrition because it is actually based on anatomy and physiology - meanwhile the 'science' of human nutrition is not. For example, nutritional research in zoos investigated what happens when chimpanzees are fed a conventional human diet – this lead to serious illness in the chimpanzees and all sorts of behavioural problems (which are of course common in western society). Meanwhile human behavioural research led by ex-chief police officer Peter Bennett at Exeter University, found that a diet with a high proportion of raw fruit and veg significantly helped in reducing behavioural problems such as stress and aggressiveness, in young offenders and young soldiers. Mineral and vitamin balances were the key.[54]

---

[53] T Colin Campbell, *The China Study*, Benbella (2005).

[54] Peter Bennett, Gail Bradley and Nicholas Bennett, *Writings on Nutrition and Behaviour*, Behavioural Health Partnership (2002).

Science is of course applied liberally across the processed food industry, with good scientists working for companies that we know are creating *seriously unhealthy foods*. And remember, there is no established western scientific discipline of health creation.

A key fact to understand is that western nutritional research has been developed by looking at the nutritional contents of what we normally eat (i.e. what foods are marketed to us) in our western culture, when we all know *the normal outcome of the modern western diet is chronic illness*. It does not consider our anatomy and physiology, or 'the ecology of nutrition'. Nutrition research, like most research, is focused on the minutiae of its subject, and includes many assumptions (e.g. about proteins and carbohydrates), which arose at a time when research was far less sophisticated. Those long-standing assumptions are largely forgotten, hidden or ignored – although they still strongly influence our thinking, research questions and cultural norms. The assumptions mean that our perception of what is 'good nutrition' is strongly influenced by out of date thinking. If nutritional research started now with a clean sheet of paper then I think it would get the right answers quite quickly. But it is starting with a sheet of paper full of old ideas and assumptions, and therefore it is often asking the wrong kinds of questions.

So the reality is that science and research is largely driven by the private sector undertaking its own research or funding university research on topics the funders select. Drug companies inevitably fund research that involves drugs - they are not going to fund research, however positive it might be, that suggests we would need few (if any) of the drugs they produce if we followed a different, more natural dietary route.

Fixed patterns of thinking and organization are common across most academic and research areas. 'Reductionism' and corporately funded research create an internal consistency that allows economists, genetic engineers, agro-chemists and politicians to justify their actions with clever but narrow perspectives, when often their arguments just don't make sense when considered within a wider view.[55] So the patterns of thinking that developed modern nutritional science are exactly the same as those that developed GMOs, toxic agrochemicals and industrial chemicals, nuclear and chemical weapons, and lots and lots and lots of pharmaceutical drugs. Nutritional science contains a lot of useful information and many powerful ideas, but that doesn't mean it has got it all 'right' (or all wrong). Drug research and weapons research start from a solid belief in drugs and weapons ... and virtually all nutritional research starts with a solid belief in cooked foods and a 'normal' western diet.

As the physicist and holistic scientist Fritjof Capra explains the reductionist problem well, and points out in his book *The Turning Point,* the significant problems of our time *"are all different facets of one and the same crisis, and that this crisis is essentially a crisis of perception."*[56]

Put another way, *if we believe in the power of science and were truly scientific in studying human health and nutrition, and perceived health and nutrition problems <u>and solutions</u> in a scientifically accurate way, most of us would be healthy by now, obviously.* Think about it.

---

[55] Reductionism involves looking narrowly at a subject, and ignoring its wider context and connections with other topics – the belief that a whole can be correctly understood by reducing it down to its known component parts, without a need to focus equally on the relationship between those parts, and external relationships.

[56] Fritjof Capra, *The Turning Point*, Bantam (1982), p.15.

Having said all that, modern nutrition is shifting in a positive direction. However, it is still largely food based rather than assimilation based. So many nutritional researchers still are not seeing the wood (health) for the trees (foods). There are very few nutritionists who are actually studying the nutrition and *nutritional relationships that naturally create vibrant health*. So, if you want to be vibrantly healthy you have to look carefully at where your nutritional advice is coming from – is it health-creating nutrition, or 'normal' nutrition?

How many nutritional researchers are vibrantly healthy? How many nutritionists are basing their opinions about eating more raw on extensive research into or experience of people following an eat more raw lifestyle? Or have any direct long term experience of eating a significant proportion of raw foods themselves? This is the best possible form of research and it is of course the one that raw foodists follow!

However, it's fair to say that the claims and dogmatism of some raw food advocates also don't necessarily help encourage research, with some naïve or outrageous claims from the movement giving scientists, the media and the public an easy opt-out that allows them to consider the lifestyle to be too wayout, crankish or extreme for serious consideration. Fortunately positive results are showing in more and more people's lives though, so the gap is closing, rather than widening. At the same time the raw food movement is maturing.

There has been virtually no funded institutional research into eating raw food diets, except for some work at Cornell University in the US and a study at Geissen University in Germany in the 1990's – which came up with very clear positive results but which was unable to gain funding to take the research further and properly promote the results.

So most nutritionists' views on an all-raw or high-raw diet is based on no direct knowledge, no experience of the subject and absolutely no research on their part – which is inconsistent if they espouse the vital importance of conclusions drawn from properly conducted research. And in this day and age it is also based on legal liability fears and peer pressure within their nutritional community. This is hardly surprising as it challenges their basic assumptions, as well as their expert reputations and their livelihoods - and their own diets of course.

If we look at other scientific fields such as anatomy and physiology we find plenty of accepted facts that contradict the conventional nutritional perspective. 'Okham's Razor' is a famous philosophical and scientific tool, which states that all things being equal, the simplest explanation will be true. With Okhams Razor in mind simple observation of nature provides a simple explanation which is that wild animals are generally totally vibrantly healthy, based on a specific physiology which is ideally suited for a specific natural diet.

So I suggest that nutritional research of two types is absolutely vital if individuals and our society are to achieve vibrant health. Firstly, well conducted, independent scientific research into *optimum health* and *optimum nutrition* which is based on physiology and starts from a clean sheet is vital. Secondly, research that is undertaken through real-life experience by individuals – which is the research you can undertake for yourself, by having a go, in an informed way, over a period of time e.g. conduct your own well informed, well designed 3 month action-research trial – like the opposite of the '*Supersize Me*' experiment (perhaps '*SuperHealth Me*' instead).

Natural health promoter Loren Lockman points out that 'God', 'Goddess', universe, nature, creation, evolution did not 'screw it up' – 'He', 'She', it or they provided us with all we need for natural health. Millions of years of experimentation and research is embodied in nature and the process of evolution that brought humans into existence – so again, in the face of a lack of a significant body of scientific research into the optimum biochemistry for the human diet, that is the source I suggest you look to.[57]

I sense that our personal understanding and our culture is approaching a scientific and social 'tipping point' in our understanding of health and nutrition. The trend is towards increased real-life research, real-life evidence and real-life understanding of the lifestyles and diets that actually create vibrant health – this is a movement you can be part of.

We're on a rising curve and it may not be long until we hit take off point, the balance tips, and the focus of our culture shifts to using its powerful formal and informal scientific resources to help create health in us as individuals and as a society. I look forward to that day!

FREQUENT AND LESS COMMON QUESTIONS AND ANSWERS

By exploring all of the frequently asked questions above in depth, over many years, I and many others have removed many of our unspoken assumptions about food and nutrition. We've found some very useful answers to those questions. From years of direct experiential research I know that it feels far 'better' to my mind-body-spirit, and 'better' for my relationship with the earth as a whole, if I eat a high proportion of raw foods. 'Better' means I feel more at ease living in this way, I feel healthier and happier, my mind is clearer and more content, my body feels better and the ripple effects feel more positive.

On a purely logical level, I know that after more than 20 years of consistently good health on a high percentage raw diet I clearly have no physiological need to eat cooked foods, meat or dairy produce. I also recognise that a high percentage raw organic diet has huge environmental benefits, because it shifts away from a diet that is associated with a great deal of environmental damage, pollution and high energy use. So to me it just feels natural to eat more raw - I find it an easier way of life. (And there's no greasy washing up or tough pan cleaning either!)

Part of the point of this book is to highlight that even within the wonderful solutions-oriented permaculture movement, a less common question is how can we design and create an optimum diet for short and long term human *and* ecological health? Let's try to answer it together.

In response to this question, the practicalities of this lifestyle, such as transitional living and 'detox', a balanced high or mainly raw diet, sprouting and juicing, all year salad beds, perennial vegetables and forest gardening are dealt with in the next section of this book.

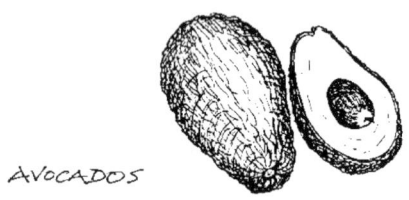
AVOCADOS

---

[57] *A Handbook for Vibrant Living – Eight Keys to Optimal Health*, Loren Lockman, Natural Designs Publishing (2001).

PART 5: THE ACTION PLAN - THE PRACTICALITIES

TRANSITIONAL LIVING

There are many routes to arrive at a change of direction, surrounding or circumstances in your life. If you want to change something, you can just stop what you are doing and change your life completely – it is possible. Some people simply stop smoking cigarettes, using cocaine, watching TV, eating wheat / gluten foods, drinking alcohol or coffee for example – all of which are addictive to varying degrees.

The same can happen when making wholesale changes in your diet – some can make rapid changes, whilst others need more time. If you do suddenly start eating a lot more raw the first one or two weeks will probably be a challenge – particularly the first 2 to 4 days, when the body starts cleaning itself out and adjust. After that you'll feel much better, although there'll be both challenges and benefits down the path.

A fairly rapid change to eating 50% raw need not be a problem for anyone. I recommend it completely, although depending on where you are starting from there may be challenges. If you are starting from a really poor diet then a change to 50% raw is a big change for your body, and it will create something of a health shock, so it's best be in touch with a friend or someone who can advise you – someone positive who has been through a similar process themselves.

A change to eating 100% raw is very different to a conventional diet, whether vegetarian or meat eating, and is very different to 50% raw. For many people it's tough to be 100% raw, although some manage it with no great problems. Beyond 50%, a planned transition to 50-70% or even 90% raw is very practical. The main thing is to feel good about what you are doing. Whether you target is 50% or 100%, if you have 'slippage' that's OK so long as you are moving in the right direction, giving your body more of a chance to create health over time.

In moving toward real health, overall giving up processed food is by far the most important first step. Do this and it will make a *big* difference to your health. In particular this includes leaving behind processed fats, processed meats, processed carbohydrates and refined sugars. Basically, the message is 'get off processed foods as fast as you can' – because that is the stuff which really messes with nature. It is chemically *unnatural* - so putting it in our bodies has a big effect on both our mind and emotions, as well as our body. Think through the effects from one generation to the next, recognising that we have had only one really full generation of highly processed food eating so far.

For example, just looking at processed fats, Dr Udo Erasmus in his excellent book and recorded talk *Fats That Kill, Fats That Heal* states that there are five 'killer fats'. These are the highly processed and cooked fats – it is shocking to discover the processes that these have typically gone through to make margarine, for example. So for anyone on a 'normal' diet one of the best first steps is to get off cooked and highly processed fats. Dr Erasmus then also explains how Omega 3 and Omega 6 fats are particularly valuable and have tremendous healing properties (i.e. flax oil, Udo's Choice oil blend, hemp oil, coconut fats).

When you get off processed foods you will be amazed and delighted at the results within two to three weeks, *particularly if you are making sure you are adding in more quality raw nutrients to your diet at the same time.* Going straight to a high fruit diet would create a heavy detox response from your body and could overload your cleansing system – so is not advisable from a poor diet. Fruit is more cleansing, which releases toxins into the blood more rapidly in the process of being flushed out. Brief dizzy spells when you stand up may happen when you come off coffee or junk food, for example – be aware of this but don't worry about it, as it's just the body getting stuff out through the blood stream and adjusting its chemical balances. It would often happen when you give up coffee, cigarettes or alcohol for example, if you've been a regular user of them, whether or not you make a change in your diet.

If you shift your diet to mainly fruit, over time the higher energy that will result from it may need some grounding through meditation or yoga - *eating more greens is really important to balance this.* To produce some of your own food, and add this to your diet change, it is particularly good to grow greens in the garden or your window boxes - start with an all-year salad garden planted up over a series of weekends, and try some sprouting indoors (see later sections and appendices for helpful advice on this).

In making these changes people naturally think 'oh, I must do this right'. However, it's important to be fair and caring to yourself, and not to feel you have to be 'perfect' – be firm and clear, but not too self-critical. Food is a very important part of peoples' lives whether they realise it or not, and making major changes can be challenging... as well as amazingly liberating.

If you *gradually eat more raw* you can't make many mistakes, although you can make a few – which this book aims to help you avoid. Frederic Paténaude's book *The Raw Secrets* is very open, honest and direct about potential raw food pitfalls. It is targeted more at those aiming for the 'all raw' diet, but there's lots of useful information in it even if you aren't aiming for that.[58] You and your body will learn as you go. The same goes for making your life more sustainable. Both these changes in your lifestyle offer long term opportunities to learn and experiment.

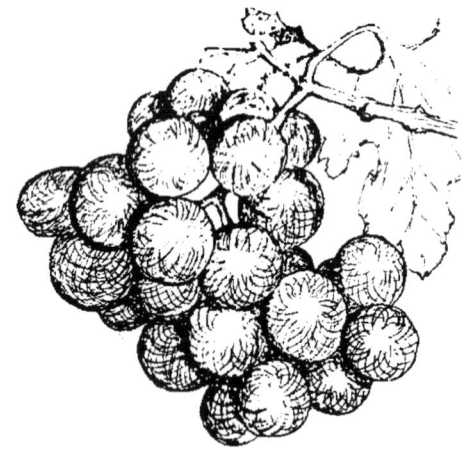

---

[58] Frederic Patenuade, *The Raw Secrets*, Raw Vegan (2002)

Creating the possibility of creating real health for yourself is the vital first step. And to bring this possibility closer to you, just starting and having a go is most important. That way you are heading in the right direction. Gaining better information is a great start. You don't have to do it overnight – you don't have to switch from cooked food one day to eating 100% raw the next day. And, you don't have to create the 'perfect' forest garden in a weekend either! Start by cutting out processed foods, whilst increasing the amount of raw food in your diet, and see what benefits you feel in the first month. The benefits may take time to become clear, and will depend on what type and proportion of raw and home grown foods you include in your diet, but normally within a couple of weeks there'll be some noticeable positive changes.

When you start to eat more raw there are five things that are really useful to know about:

1. *Fruit-only breakfasts/mornings are a great way to start the day.* Also, eat fruit on its own and 30 minutes or more before your meal rather than after, because it is digested quickly and easily (half an hour if it is ripe). This avoids bad food combinations which causes a ferment (i.e. wind/gas). Apples are a bit of an exception, as they tend to combine well with leaf and vegetable salads, although not with starchy cooked foods.

2. *Drink fresh green juices or vegetable juices and consume the highest quality fats* - this will really make a difference. Mixed fruit and veg juices are also great.

3. *Develop an understanding of food combining.* Your body produces different types of digestive juices for digestion of starches and proteins, and certain foods combine well, whilst others combine badly; particularly starches and proteins, or starches and sweet fruit. Poor combining creates fermentation in the digestive system, which prevents digestion. Mixing green veg (e.g. lettuce, kale) and non-starchy vegetables (e.g. cauli) with protein foods (seeds) *or* starches is a good combination – combining protein *and* starches is a bad combination.

4. *Start your main meals with a raw salad*, at least for the first few mouthfuls - use cold pressed oils in dressings and freshly squeezed lemon juice.

5. Understand that *the first part of your transition is a cleansing process*, and is something you can design and manage, and be thankful for.

The nitty-gritty of good and bad food combinations is that there are three bacterial processes which can happen in the digestive system: digestion, fermentation and putrefaction – two of these processes are 'bad' and one is 'good'. Digestion is the good process through which we assimilate nutrition, and is dependent on good bacteria (lacto-bacteria) in the digestive system. Fermentation (of sugars and starches) and putrefaction (of proteins) happen when unhealthy and badly combined foods are eaten, which are then broken down by bacteria in the digestive system but in these cases producing toxic excretions.

The food combining issue can seem a little confusing at first but it is easy to get the hang of once you start looking at your meals in terms of the food groups in the following food combining chart. An important point to note is that essentially there are 13 good combinations, but only 3 bad combinations. Focus on avoiding the 3 bad combinations to simplify things.

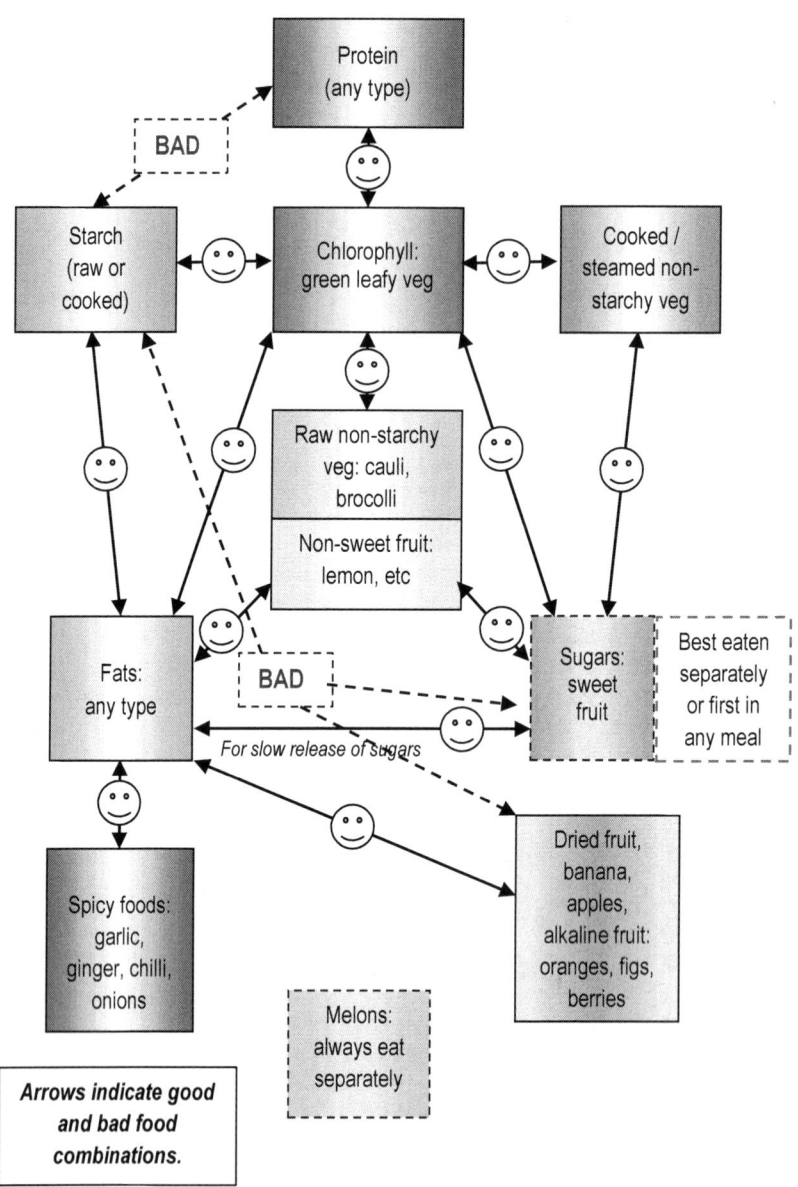

A Basic Food Combining Chart

Adapted from diagram in *The Sunfood Diet Success System*, by David Wolfe.

There's a lot of focus on foods. But what is equally *essential* is to focus on your body – because nutritional health is a direct interaction between your food and your body. In particular your nutritional health depends on:

a) your body's ability to *assimilate* nutrition;
b) its ability to *get rid of* what's harmful to it – to de-toxify.

So if your digestive system is clogged up with undigested starches and proteins, cooked fats and other food debris then it is difficult for the nutrition in the food to make its way into the body. Eating the best foods is far better than eating the worst foods, but to get the best results you need to *clean up your digestive system as well*, and help your body shift stuff which may be stored all over the place. Understanding these two aspects of nutritional health allows you to move to a higher level of thinking in relation to creating health.

Fortunately the best raw plant foods will help in both these aspects of healthy nutrition, as they help to get rid of some of the harmful substances as well as providing good quality nutrients in a form that is easy to assimilate. Just having fresh juice for several days – 'a juice fast' – is a very good way to accelerate this, and often people really enjoy it after the first day or so. Fully cleansing out the system needs more radical action like herbal cleanses, longer fasts or a full programme of colonics. [59] It is not natural for this 'gunk' to be in your body, so your body does not have a natural mechanism to get rid of it. It's tough stuff to shift! [60]

Exercise is also hugely beneficial, particularly yoga, aerobic exercise, tai chi and so on. Dance is great too, and using a rebounder (mini-trampolene) also brings excellent results.

PRACTICAL ACTIONS

1. Seek balance and don't become obsessed about raw foods or food in general, thinking you have to be a 'perfect' raw fooder. You are making positive changes, improving the chain of cause-and-effect within your body and the wider world. Food is not everything in life, by any means!
2. Understand the nature and effects of foods that are heavy and slow, which take a lot of energy to digest, making you feel sleepy because you don't have the energy to digest them and stay awake at the same time. To blast away this sleepiness we habitually use five main stimulants to keep us awake in the short term, but which all have harmful long term effects: caffeine, sugar, nicotine, salt and excess protein. If you drop the heavy, sleepy-fog-inducing foods for lighter foods, then it's easier to drop the (addictive) stimulants.
3. Get to know the foods that are cleansing, life giving and energising. Get a feel in your body for the biology and bio-chemistry of foods.
4. Get to know the alkalizing foods and acidifying foods, and shift towards 80% alkaline foods.

---

[59] The Arise and Shine and Ejuva herbal cleanses are widely used, and I've met many people who've had great results from them;

[60] See the classic *Colon Health* by Dr Norman Walker, Norwalk Press (1995) – and for information on digestive system cleansing see Sura retreats at www.suradetox.com

5. Study life, natural processes and evolution. What I mean is using your own observation and experience to get a really deep feel for nature's 'innate intelligence'.
6. Fully taste the foods you eat and really listen to your body, because it will tell you a lot if you really listen; allow it to tell you which foods feel like they will create health, and listen.
7. Make yourself plans and then put your plan into action: (a) for changes in your foods, (b) to cleanse your body and digestive system and (c) for physical activities to aid blood and lymphatic circulation, cleansing and breathing.

MAKING THE TRANSITION

Many raw educators emphasise that foods don't cure anything at all. The body itself cures everything. Every organism is self-healing, and good health is the natural condition for a body. As Loren Lockman says: *'what we can do, is to provide the body with the optimal conditions in which to heal itself'*.[61] If we learn this individually, in our families and communities, and as a society then excellent health will be the natural result.

Dr Joel Robbins suggests starting simply by adding more raw foods into your diet, without worrying about changing much else. Gradually you will then be drawn to eat more raw foods by what Dr Robbins calls the body's 'innate intelligence'.[62] In this way he even found that his fanatical enjoyment of hot and spicy Mexican food disappeared without any loss of pleasure or satisfaction from his diet.

Frederic Paténaude on the other hand emphasizes that all bad habits are bad habits. Smaller bad habits still prevent you from being healthy and can encourage constant slippage. If someone wants to stop smoking, slowly cutting down from 40-a-day to five cigarettes per day is a big and positive change – but it is still very different to giving up completely, and is a difference that prevents the really big benefits from happening.

If you prefer to make more rapid changes, and if this move is well informed and supported, it will bring the benefits of change more quickly, although it will also intensify the symptoms of the basic cleansing process. It means getting things that limit your health out of the way more quickly and can be good if you enjoy a challenge – physical, mental, emotional and/or spiritual.

So, one thing must be made clear: to reach an optimum level of health it is a question of a) eating whatever the best diet for health may seem to be, and b) getting rid of the unhealthy material in your body that will get in the way of better nutrition creating optimal health.

Put another way:

The nutrition your body will be able to receive and work with = what it is able to assimilate + what is fed into it.

What your body is able to take in depends on the state of your digestive system, as well as your body's cleansing and rebuilding systems. For optimal health all these parts have to be addressed to create a healthy whole.

---

[61] Loren Lockman, *A Handbook for Vibrant Living – Eight Keys to Optimal Health*, Natural Designs Publishing (2001).

[62] Dr Joel Robbins CD, *Health Through Nutrition* (Health & Wellness Center)

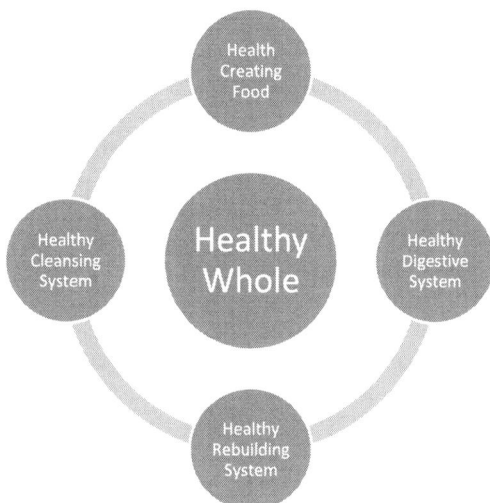

For most people, advancing to roughly 50% raw can be done quickly and then beyond that a gradual transition suits many, because you'll have a gentler release of the toxins in the body, easing the physical and emotional reactions to detoxification. Keeping the exercise plan and steady cleansing process going through this time is really important. The challenge is to remember all this and *know that you are making good headway* when you are in the midst of a pounding headache, feeling irritated, with a furry tongue, *all caused by your body's success and intelligence in naturally kicking out the unwanted rubbish!*

The speed of this process depends on what you are eating and how much cleansing you have already done. If you are 50% raw but still eating 50% junk / processed food, wheat, meat or dairy you are still not eating a healthy enough diet to get the biggest benefits.

A vital factor is how you feel about making the change. If you feel clear, enthusiastic and positive or determined then it will be easier. If you think you should change but don't really want to it will be more difficult, and less fun. So *know where you really want to be, enjoy the journey and have a clear goal*. Connecting with others on a similar path is also often a big help. This all helps support and strengthen the real health possibility that you are creating for yourself.[63]

Set yourself some monthly targets or daily targets. For example in *The New Raw Energy* Leslie and Susannah Kenton suggest having weekly 'apple days', where you only have apples during the morning initially, and then just apples for a whole day once a week.[64] Apples are excellent foods for such an approach because they are so well balanced (make sure they are ripe and ideally organic though). Another option is to have one or more all raw days each week.

---

[63] Dr Joel Robbins CD/download, *Attitudes to Health* (Health & Wellness Center) is very helpful.
[64] Leslie and Susannah Kenton, *The New Raw Energy*, Vermillion (1994).

Fruit-only breakfasts and mornings immediately demonstrate the time and energy saving benefits of eating more raw. I started (in autumn going into winter of all times) by switching to a fruit-only breakfast and having a salad, with sprouted organic seeds or pulses for lunch. In the evening I had another salad, and added steamed potatoes or cooked millet half way through. And I must point out that to me salad means something much more interesting and enjoyable than just lettuce, cucumber and tomato! It doesn't take much effort to experiment and learn the huge and delicious variety of things you can use to create a salad – especially if you grow some rocket, parsley, peltaria, chives and a variety of other greens and herbs for yourself. Just grow 5 different greens as a start, add them to your salad each day, and you'll feel and taste the difference it makes – your 5 a day salad mix. (See the Recipes section for more info!)

So in the early part of my journey into the hidden world of healthy nutrition, without me really noticing, my body's desire for the starchy foods disappeared during the winter, and when Spring arrived I found it easier to grab a bag of apples and some nuts and dried fruit for lunch than to make a salad. So, without making a decision to do so I switched from two thirds salad and one third fruit to one third salad and two thirds fruit – which felt both natural and great!

This practical-first-steps approach is also important for moving to a more ecological and humane way of life. The process of change itself must be sustainable – so it needs to feel good to you. And this is where the pressure to be 'all raw' often fails, or can cause emotional difficulties. So to ease your path you may want to go on some workshops or courses, or contact networks and know where to find information *and support* from people you share common ideals and motivations with (many helpful contacts are detailed in the Appendices section).

Allow change to happen by recognising that the world and your life is a constant flow of change. Movement is always happening although at times it may seem slow – at other times it may feel like a roller-coaster ride! We all make choices and base them on our experience, our feelings and the information we have to hand. So there is no intention here of forcing anyone to change their diet – the choice is yours. However, I do humbly suggest that you base your choices on good information, your own experience and careful observation over a long enough time. Do your own research by having a go, explore the subject, and keep your eyes, your heart and your mind open while considering the important issues in your life.

In nature, the one thing you can be sure of being constant is perpetual change - often this is a stable and steady form of change that you hardly notice, whilst at other times it's more disruptive. And often disruptive change can turn out to be very positive, although it might feel really tough when it's happening. Try to work with this principle of natural change coming in different forms, depending on the circumstances. Unless you put yourself in an all or mainly raw environment, for a lot of people, taking a larger number of smaller steps over time will lead to more stable change in the long term than a small number of big steps in a short time. Once this is accepted, you can look towards making steady conscious changes in what you eat, in your exercise, your cleansing plan and in how you obtain your food, and be happy with the idea that this will take time to work through. You can plan, design and manage it, including setting yourself some positive milestones to celebrate - you can also get unexpected adventures along the way. It's a journey.

DETOXIFICATION AND CLEANSING: A NATURAL PROCESS

For most of us 'Detox' is part and parcel of creating the possibility of significantly improved health. It is a natural detoxification or cleansing process that the body initiates when it has the opportunity (the energy and resources) to do so.

Another way of looking at it is that if we eat a normal western diet then 'toxification' of the body (i.e. a build-up of toxins) is inevitable and 'naturally' happens gradually over a lifetime. *So eating a typical western diet and following a typical western lifestyle we cannot actually avoid toxification.* This means that genuine health (which is different to fitness) cannot be achieved without some kind of de-toxication process i.e. when you eat health-creating foods (rather than illness creating foods), giving your body the chance to clear out the toxification that's stored in it. This happens much faster when just water and no food is coming in – this is fasting.

Detoxification is usually like having a heavy cold, because it's your body's opportunity to clear out some gunk and mucous! Early on, a detox may also include some bowel clearance as your body flushes out stored toxins that it has decided it is now safe to release. If you know what's happening you can welcome this, knowing that your body is using it's innate intelligence to create health, even though you're likely to feel a bit rough – or sometimes very rough!

Detox or cleansing symptoms can include:

- Fuzzy headedness or headaches (sometimes severe): flushing out toxins in the blood affecting the brain.
- Clogged up or running nose: release of unwanted mucous.
- Sore throat: a sensitive area affected by toxins released into the blood.
- Mouth ulcers: release of toxins through the sensitive skin of the mouth.
- Weariness and a Foggy Brain: toxins in the blood affecting the muscles and energy diverted to cleansing the body, making less available to the brain.
- Itchy skin, Spots and Skin conditions: toxins and 'bad fats' coming out through the pores in the skin, the body's largest organ.
- Irritability: released toxins affecting thinking, feelings and moods.
- Unpleasant breath and body odours: toxins released through skin and breath.

Sounds horrible, eh? I'd say 'yes and no'! Actually it is your body doing a great job of dumping unwanted stuff, which could do much greater harm to you in the long term than you'll experience in the detox/cleansing process. These are the physical and emotional effects of a bunch of unnatural chemicals (from things you've eaten) being released into the bloodstream and lymphatic system. With toxins coming into the expulsion system the natural response of the body is to want to rest because it needs to divert energies away from its normal activities to cope with the extra work of ridding itself of these toxins. So weariness is normal. It's the body telling you "rest me, I want to use my energy to get rid of this stuff!" Plenty of sleep or dozing helps cleansing because it gives the body a good period of rest from eating, and takes your mind off the detox symptoms. Keep yourself entertained and distracted. And if you don't feel like eating don't eat, just drink water or fresh juice – but not for more than a day or two at this early stage, if you've come from a typical diet or especially a high junk/processed food diet.

However, sometimes at the same time as experiencing these unpleasant effects there can also be positive feelings of exhilaration that result from the body's removal of toxins. So there can be weariness mixed with a strong desire to have vigorous exercise, to walk, run or do sport or yoga, because activity helps get the blood pumping and to improve the release of toxins through the lymphatic system and organs, including pushing things out through the skin by sweating. Your body knows this, so sometimes creates this desire to be active to help pump out the rubbish.

Many people concerned with health, and not just raw fooders, understand that we have to go through this cleansing process if we want to strive for real health – because we have to shift the toxins that pose a long term threat to our health. Fasting, saunas, sweat lodges, colonics and herbal cleanses are other valuable ways of stimulating the detox and cleansing process. However, unless you're fairly well cleaned out already it is not advisable to combine all these together - although colonics or enemas generally work well with other cleansing processes, such as juice fasting. The immune system is the driving force behind the detox and cleansing process. So all these techniques are ways to strengthen or stimulate the immune system and its innate intelligence. They are ways of helping along the process of getting things out of the way so that the body and immune system can then get on with their job of creating real health.

If someone has a lot of toxins stored in their body and their detox or cleansing is too rapid, then it is possible for it to have some dangerous effects. However, these are only possible if someone takes an extreme approach to detoxing, such as going straight into a water only fast straight from a junk food diet. Such an extreme approach can lead to a huge release of toxins into the blood if you've been eating a lot of junk. This can create an unnaturally high toxic release which overloads the body's organs and filters, and which can then pose some dangers, including to the brain. Such effects would only happen if you go quickly from a very toxic diet into a serious fast, which I strongly do not recommend.

If you are well informed, or have contact with others with knowledge and experience, and if you maintain a good balance of vitamins and minerals, particularly fresh green vegetables, the benefits of detoxification greatly outweigh any short term unpleasant effects. Two good sources of information and motivation to have at hand before or during a detox are the book *Raw Emotions* by Angela Stokes, and the movie *Fat, Sick and Nearly Dead*.

Detox symptoms can be stopped either by stopping the detox process itself, by diverting energy and resources away from it, or by encouraging it to its natural conclusion. To encourage and assist it you should drink plenty of liquid, either spring water, fresh raw juices or distilled water to help flush the toxins through the body – carrot, beetroot, apple and celery based juices are really good for this. Well informed short fasts (e.g. 2-3 days) will also accelerate this cleansing process. Using plenty of fresh greens (and/or food state mineral supplements) is also important to help replenish the body, particularly if you are coming from a diet that has been very unhealthy.[65] However, going back to eating more normally (i.e. some cooked foods, such as steamed or lightly boiled vegetables) will also normally stop the detox process where it is. The body's 'innate intelligence' will then take it up again when it feels ready – if you give it the chance.

---

[65] For example, see www.marineminerals.com

Fasting is a powerful route to detoxification. Fasting is used in many spiritual traditions because it challenges the mind, body and spirit, so that the faster can draw understanding and strength – and also cleans the mind, body and spirit, allowing a clearer and deeper spiritual connection in its latter stages and beyond. It is essential to be well informed and well prepared before entering into a fast, as this can rapidly release many stored toxins into the body. The body needs to be in good shape to deal with the kind of cleansing a major fast can bring on. Do not go straight into fasting from a very poor diet - you are better off *not* fasting until you have shifted to eating a healthier diet for a while e.g. at least a couple of months. The key message is to read and consult others about it first, and make sure you've got others around you, or do a supervised fast. Arnold Ehret's excellent book *Rational Fasting* is probably the most straight-forward, has been a best seller for years and is also inexpensive.[66] After curing himself of an 'incurable' disease through fasting, followed by many years of fasting research, and unparalleled personal experience for a westerner (including two scientifically supervised fasts of around 50 days) Professor Ehret recommended *regular short fasts* of three days to one week, but did not recommend the very long fasts which he undertook himself earlier in his life.

Many raw foods websites and networks supply good books with excellent information on fasting. Although many friends a lot of fasting experience, it is one area of my transition to an eat more raw lifestyle that I would change with hindsight, because I didn't come into contact with fasting information early in my raw path – looking back, perhaps the focus of those around me, and of the FRESH Network at the time (in the 1990's) was more on food, and less on cleansing. The movement didn't have such a balanced view of the essentials of active detoxification as it tends to have now (although I remember some people were very aware of it).

My observation of others has shown me that sensible fasting can really help. If I had known more people with fasting experience earlier on or read more on the subject earlier I am sure I would have done some short fasts earlier in my transition to raw foods, or used some herbal cleanses (I did do a ton of juicing!). Apart from the cleansing benefits, fasting also provides the body and emotions with confidence to break unhealthy patterns of emotional eating and habitual eating, which often kick in even when no nutrition is actually needed by the body. Breaking such unhealthy patterns is really helpful, particularly for emotional eaters, and is an important area for anyone to work on. Stimulants often suppress emotions. So when these stimulants are reduced or removed powerful feelings often come to the surface, and even if we didn't seem to be emotional eaters before, we can fall into this trap as we cleanse.[67] A small amount of emotional eating is almost inevitable for most of us, and won't necessarily do us harm at all. However, if it becomes out of hand then we'll have replaced one set of unhealthy habits for another.

To summarise, the key point to remember is that during the transition to a health creating diet and lifestyle cleansing is as important as eating well. Remember to *tackle both of these interrelated issues*, but also make sure you *do not become obsessed with either*.

---

[66] Arnold Ehret, *Rational Fasting*, Ehret Literature Publishing Company, Fifteenth Edition (1994) – a book which has been consistently in print since 1926 because it is such a good source of information.

[67] Angela Stokes' *Raw Emotions*, Monarch Publishing (2009) is incredibly helpful in this area.

OTHER ISSUES: CLIMATIC, SEASONAL AND LOCAL FOODS

Eating foods from your climate makes a difference to your body's temperature tolerance. Eating tropical fruit makes the body think it's in a tropical climate. Meanwhile eating foods that are appropriate to the season will help your body to be in tune with the grander cycles of nature. So eating summer crops shipped in from the opposite side of the world during winter can be confusing and chilling for your body. Eating food from your own climate, from your own patch, means the body knows where it's at temperature and climate wise, as well as reducing packaging and food miles. In a temperate climate this means more of an emphasis on greens,, stored fruit and veg, and nuts in winter, and less light juicy fruit. Sourcing local foods also means direct support for your local community and economy, reducing the 'leaky barrel', where so much money flows out from already weakened local economies into the over-dominant global economy.[68]

Apples and other fruit from the other side of the world, or veg flown in from another hemisphere should be avoided because of their massive air miles – so, if you can, choose avocados or oranges from Spain rather South Africa for example (if you're reading this in Britain or Europe!). Think about this in relation to Zones A (local) to G (global) set out in Part Three - and work out a balance that is sane, humane and sustainable – try and keep basic foods to mainly within the bioregion, with more exotic foods mainly being from within your global region.

MINERALS AND CLEANSING

Trace minerals are important. So, as raw vegetables are the best sources of minerals, fresh green /vegetable juices or high quality food state supplements can help a lot. David Wolfe promotes the vital role of mineral rich foods because of the mineral-depleted soils our foods are grown in, and because minerals are needed to support the cleansing process. He stresses foods that are especially good providers of key minerals in their natural, organically bound form:

- Celery has some of the highest levels of natural, organically bound salts, and is therefore a very important food.
- Chromium is in cinnamon, magnesium is in saffron, and silicon, a very important mineral, is found in very high levels in horsetail, nettles, hemp leaves and romaine lettuce.

Gaining information on these trace nutrients is a choice. Personally, I'm a bit lazy in these matters and tend not to worry about the specific minerals in particular foods – I just tend to eat a good variety of fresh, home/local grown green vegetables, fruit and wild foods (generally greens, some fruits), knowing from study and from experience that this diversity and balance will naturally give me what I need. This gives me far more of the best health building minerals, vitamins and enzymes than I ever had before I was raw. For others, such as pregnant or nursing mothers or city dwellers with less easy access to high quality greens, using high quality food-state supplements makes a lot of sense (particularly minerals e.g. Marine Minerals).

---

[68] The New Economics Foundation (London) work on 'the leaky barrel' and other work is an excellent source of information on healthy local economies.

ACID / ALKALINE BALANCE

A core aim of healthy eating is to create a slightly alkaline body as this is the natural state for vibrant health. Aiming for 80% alkaline foods is a good guide. The 'normal' western diet is highly acid forming, with lots of grains, meat, refined sugar and dairy being the main causes. The body can survive if it is acid - but if your blood becomes acid you die very quickly. Having an acid body increases physical stress and emotional tension – so if you look around, you'll see that an acid body often creates an acid personality. The body struggles with the typical diet, maintaining the blood's alkalinity by a) draining the body of its alkaline minerals, and b) raising acidity elsewhere in the body i.e. in the stomach or colon, which then causes ulcers or ulcerative colitis. This is all it can do because it doesn't have mineral rich, alkalising foods coming into the body. Dr Joel Robbins' *Health Through Nutrition* CD's explain all this particularly well.[69]

What is important is a food's effect on the body. Some foods that people think of as acid, such as ripe citrus fruit, in fact alkalize the body. Raw plant foods mainly have an alkaline effect, while foods typically in a western diet such as grains, refined sugar, fish, meat, poultry, shellfish, cheese, milk, and salt mainly acidify the body. And there is plenty of evidence suggesting that many of our society's major illnesses are strongly linked to an acidifying diet. Our ability to fight illness and disease (our immune response) is also directly linked to acid-alkaline balance.

In an acid state, the body craves 'quick-hits' in a dire attempt to balance its acidity and stimulate the body, and those that are easily available in our culture are the powerful alkaloids of coffee, tobacco and drugs, which have this effect. But after their immediate hit, their net effect is very much to maintain acidity, through the chain of reactions they cause in the body and appetite. Understanding this part of the cycle of cravings can help to break that cycle - if you eat more highly alkalising foods your cravings for these addictive acid-causing alkaloids will reduce.

An acid body degenerates the cells, because acids eat away at things. We need acids in our body, for example to help break down our food - but the balance of alkaline to acid has to be around 80% alkaline to 20% acid if we are to maintain true vital health. Dairy and meat, coffee and drugs (both medicinal and recreational) are some of the most extremely acidifying things our bodies have to cope with. Raw foods that are acid forming and which therefore need to be eaten in moderation, and eaten with alkalising foods, are unsoaked/unsprouted nuts, grains and seeds, and avocados. Soaked grains, nuts and seeds (soaked overnight, and then drained and rinsed) are less acid forming than if they are unsoaked. Green leafy vegetables and wild greens are the most alkaline of foods; celery and cucumbers are also excellent. Other alkaline fruits if they are ripe (and remember many supermarket foods are not ripe) include figs, sun dried and unsalted black olives, grapefruit, lemon – which is a great alkaliser - and ripe citrus fruit in general, grapes with seeds, and papaya. Wild and organic fruit is definitely best, while overly sweet, hybridised fruits are more acid forming because of the unnaturally high levels of sugars.

So 'eat more raw' = 'eat more alkaline'. And how to make the change? Well, try storing all your alkalizing foods together to start with, so you know that you mainly need to take foods from that box, container, cupboard or shelf. Tricks like this can make the changes easier.

---

[69] Visit http://ejuva.com/store/Digital-Downloads.html - any Dr Joel Robbins talk will be a great investment

SODIUM / POTASSIUM BALANCE

Sodium and potassium are vital for maintaining healthy cells, because they determine the osmotic pressure of the fluids both inside and outside the cells, which in turn determines the cells' ability to pass unwanted materials out through these liquids. If the osmotic pressure is wrong then the cell cannot get the undesirables out, leading to cellular degeneration over time. Most western diets are high in inorganic sodium (i.e. table/rock salt) and low in potassium, and for this reason our cells / bodies are unable to cleanse themselves in a healthy way.

If you can get the sodium / potassium and acid / alkaline balances right in a diet, then you will make great strides to natural health and vitality. These balances are highlighted in many nutrition and natural health books, because they are key factors in maintaining the healthy cells in your organs, blood, nervous system – all over your body. And if you keep your cells healthy, you keep your body healthy.

To keep things simple, you need to know what foods are good for getting your (organically bound) sodium and potassium balance right. Most western diets have excessive sodium, so often eating more potassium foods helps, and cutting out table salt and highly salted foods. David Wolfe's books *The Sunfood Diet Success System* and *Eating for Beauty*, provide much detail on the mineral contents of various foods.[70] To get good levels of potassium you need to eat more green leafy vegetables, celery, most fruits especially apples, avocados, bananas, dates, durian, persimmon or kaki (with seeds), and pumpkin, as well as dried fruit; raisins with seeds, prunes and apricots. Macadamia nuts and sunflower seeds are also good potassium sources.

You also need to make sure your organic sources of sodium are healthy sources. This means green leafy vegetables, and particularly celery, kale and spinach, with seaweed being another good source. Fortunately celery, kale and spinach are all easy to grow in a wide range of climates, so you can create your own organic sources of these minerals quite quickly.

In his book *Raw Secrets* Frederic Paténaude even states simply and clearly that salt is actually toxic to the body: 'Salt kills life which is why we preserve foods in salt – it prevents living activity from occurring. It is an anti-biotic, which means 'anti-life'… It causes the body to retain water in order to dilute the salt in the tissues, and to prevent harming the cells.' Technically table salt/rock salt is not a food because it provides no nutrition at all. Just so you know!

Salt is often a tough thing to give up, so allow yourself time by eating more of the naturally sodium rich foods, so that your salt-cravings go down. Use more seaweeds instead of salt, and do not over-indulge on olives! Make sure they are organic and rinse them in unsalted water before eating them. Switch to high quality sea-salt (which is high in many other minerals) if you continue using salt, and start using less than half as much as you are used to, have regular meals without any salt at all (i.e. fruit meals), or only add herb salt or sea salt in to a salad when you have eaten most of it already.[71]

---

[70] David Wolfe, *Sunfood Diet Success System*, Nature's First Law (2000) and *Eating for Beauty*, Sunfood Nutrition (2002).

[71] Sea Salt can be much more local than salt hacked out of the poor old Himalaya, shipped around the world, emitting yet more carbon in the process.

TAKE CARE OF YOURSELF IN THE SHORT & LONG TERM: MAINTAINING BALANCE

Health educator Loren Lockman suggests that there are different levels of health:

- *Transitional health:* with many positive effects including higher energy, generally feeling much better, noticeable physical improvements, etc.
- *Vibrant health:* it will take time to achieve truly vibrant health – it follows from transitional health if the right conditions are maintained.

Transitional health will feel very good in comparison with 'normal' health – it is the necessary step towards vibrant health. Both states depend on what nutrition you *are able to assimilate* (i.e. take in through your digestive system), as much as *what you eat*.

Assimilation is central to a healthy diet. Over-eating, too much fat and protein, and stress all inhibit assimilation. Being relaxed, eating an alkaline diet and when hungry rather than to satisfy appetite and cravings, will ensure you are on the path towards improved assimilation. Taking action to clean out the digestive system, through diet, colonics or herbal cleanses will accelerate this further, and it will really help you take care of yourself in the long term.

The short and long term effects of an eat more raw lifestyle tend to be very positive although they depend on each person's starting point in health, diet, life experiences and emotional patterns. Sensitivity to taste and smell, and in other areas is a common experience of eating more raw. In this area, there are several issues to be aware of:

- *Emotional sensitivity* often rises, with one's 'senses' (from first to sixth and beyond!) generally becoming more 'sensitive'. So when feelings arise they are clearer and more direct. Try not to be disconcerted by this. Emotions are a natural pointer to situations of physical or emotional discomfort and imbalance, or comfort and balance. So be aware that you may become more sensitive, and ensure that your lifestyle and/or circle of friends can be supportive of this.
- *Sensitivity to pollution*, particularly air-borne pollution – this was very obvious to me when I first went raw living in the city of Leicester (UK). Cycling to work each morning, I found it increasingly difficult to tolerate the effects of the traffic pollution on my throat and on how I felt generally. My throat became mildly sore within a few minutes of cycling in traffic; this would gradually disappear over half-an-hour or so, once I had arrived at work.
- *Sensitivity to noise and the urban lifestyle*. This will depend on how much raw you eat. Eating all or mainly raw you could become less tolerant of the noise and bustle of large towns and cities, and feel drawn to a more peaceful lifestyle. However, like everyone else most raw fooders still live in towns and cities, so for many the health and energy benefits they feel can give them more 'get up and go' and more joy in life even in an urban lifestyle.
- *Sensitivity to other diets and lifestyles*. If you eat all or mainly raw this can be tough, as you can start to think that everyone else's diet is almost insane, not even 'food'. This is the *'Why can't they see?'* syndrome and is not an uncommon reaction to many kinds of revelations. This often happens when people think or feel they have found 'THE' answer, and it can be common for raw foodies to think raw food is 'THE' answer. Beware of this because it will normally lead to feeling very frustrated when others 'just don't get it'.

If you get involved in the raw movement you may quickly find that those who see raw foods as THE single answer tend to be less balanced than those who see a bigger picture. Raw food, healthy living or permaculture fundamentalism may be more positive, more healthy and more sustainable – but they are not balanced. The most impressive advocates of any movement or philosophy are those who express compassion, tolerance and understanding, with strong inner self-confidence and certainty. Such people tend not to preach - they get on and do it. Whatever you believe or eat, it is normally *not* very effective if you go around trying to convert everyone, and being intolerant of other people's diets. Preaching, arguing or attacking the diet or lifestyle of others will lead to an understandably defensive response to your attack. Allow others to have their own revelations in their own time, like you, rather than cramming it down their throat. Demonstrate the benefits of a healthier diet, by experiment and by example. To provide more information and healthier choices to people, listen to them and hear their needs, be yourself and be comfortable living your own life - the more at ease you are with your own diet and lifestyle, the more people will be open, interested and inquiring about these things. If someone opens a door towards you, the harder you push on it the more firmly it may close in your face.

Sometimes, when people discover the seriousness of the world's social, ecological and health/sickness problems, anger can emerge, along with other emotions. If someone's life experience has made them susceptible to anger or aggression (which sadly is fairly common in our society) then eating more raw may make them more sensitive. Anger can arise in the detox process, and can be an understandable response to the kinds of 'crimes against nature and humanity' we see in the world, but if that anger becomes aggression it worsens the problem. If anger emerges as you make changes in your life, then work to channel that anger positively, in ways that are firm but not aggressive or violent, either physically or emotionally.[72] If this happens, then *focus on alkalizing your diet*. It may be easier said than done, but rather than trying to suppress or block anger, try to direct it positively and transform it.

On the whole, *an eat more raw lifestyle is much more likely to reduce aggression than increase it* particularly if focuses on raising the alkalinity of the diet. Stress, anger and tension can arise from a 'normal' diet because it lacks key nutrients and trace elements. Research on aggressive and dysfunctional behaviour in military trainees and criminals by Peter Bennett of The Behavioural Health Partnership found that significant improvement in diet lead to significant improvements in behaviour.[73] Dealing with anger can be challenge whether you are a coming from being a meat eater or vegan. Many angry vegans who've started eating more raw have found they feel less aggressive about animal rights issues, whilst feeling equally strongly, and being at least as effective in their campaigning – they see that violent attitudes towards human animals are no better than violent attitudes towards other animals. Highly processed foods and junk food, even if it's vegan, is very acidifying – it aggravates the body as a whole, including the nerves and emotions. So alkalizing the diet is a key strategy to reduce anger, although I'm not suggesting it's enough on its own to remove the anger.

---

[72] A great booklet to help you understand your anger is *What's Making You Angry*, by Klein and Gibson, Puddle Dancer Press, from www.NonviolentCommunication.com or www.liferesources.co.uk

[73] Peter Bennett et al, *Writings on Nutrition and Behaviour*, BHP (2002).

The other extreme is also possible. If you already feel alienated in a world which is often violent, harsh and aggressive to one's senses then eating a lot more raw food is probably not going to lessen that feeling, although for some it might. *Raw Emotions* (2009), by Angela Stokes, was the first book to confront many of these emotional issues head on.[74] As such it is a very important and very welcome book to emerge from the raw food world.

A 50%+ raw lifestyle may take you to a point where you feel desperate to change your living situation to one that is more in harmony with your senses, your true nature, and to be with similar people. The sense of desperation will not be pleasant if you are isolated, but if you make positive changes in your living situation that desperation can be replaced with something much more pleasant - perhaps you might find a peaceful home in nature or in a community of raw fooders.[75] This is one of the points about combining the natural health and sustainability perspectives. Your whole lifestyle situation needs to be looked at, with diet as just a part of it.

Discovering raw food nutrition, sustainability or permaculture can open your eyes to many things. What I see and feel is that diet and lifestyle is part of a huge web of inter-connected effects. Changing your diet and lifestyle will have very significant effects. This includes reactions to other people, what they say and how they behave, and to your own lifestyle and the world around you. Finding a more positive diet and lifestyle is important but do not expect instant answers to all your problems, or all the problems of the world. Whatever route you take you will experience change, and that can be fascinating, fulfilling and fun in itself. Like many things in life, the best results often emerge over time through persistence and commitment - like a maturing garden. Adopt an approach that takes care of yourself on many levels, not just the physical, through times of change. A challenging vision can be reached if we consistently take practical, achievable steps on the path toward that vision.

Ask yourself:
1. Where am I now and where am I heading?
2. What's my realistic vision of where I *really* want to be?
3. What are my first practical steps towards getting there?
4. How can I take those steps and when?

These days many mystics and scientists say the same thing about the nature of nature; that chaos reigns (although this is not 'chaos' in a negative sense). Getting a feel for nature and chaos will give you a stronger sense of how positive changes in your own lifestyle will effect positive and often subtle changes in the wider whole. The true nature of chaos is an ever moving complexity of inter-related effects, which includes a fundamental degree of uncertainty. It's not necessarily without structure – every tree is an example of *chaos*, which also embodies a natural *structure* in its trunk, branches and twigs. So any major change, evolution or revolution, in your lifestyle, or in a whole society, can throw out a whole range of unexpected effects. So if you do make rapid changes in your life, do 'expect the unexpected', as they say.

---

[74] Angela Stokes, *Raw Emotions*, Monarch Publishing (2009) e-book/paperback from www.rawreform.com
[75] Sadly there are few of these – maybe it's time for you to take part in creating one? I did, so you can!

CHRONIC ILLNESSES AND MAJOR HEALTH CHALLENGES

Personal stories of people who have overcome chronic illnesses, or major health challenges, using diet are common - normally alongside a positive mindset, and a belief that they can overcome or significantly reduce the challenge they faced. Many raw food books deal with this healing aspect of raw foods, so I am not going into it in depth here. Although, within the raw foods and healing nutrition movement an all raw or high percentage raw diet has been seen to help many people with the following serious conditions:

- Various cancers (particularly green juice / wheatgrass have been found to be highly beneficial, also other fresh vegetable/fruit juices) – supporting the immune system to help fight the cancer; feeding the body with vibrant, alive and nutrient rich foods.
- Heart disease and high blood pressure – replacing unhealthy fats with healthy fats, supplying key minerals and vitamins for healthy heart and blood system function, reducing acidity and raising alkalinity - cleansing the arteries and the blood itself.
- Obesity and weight problems – see Angela's story in Part Four.
- Diabetes – balancing sugars, carbohydrates and the critical chemistry involved in their management and release.
- Chronic kidney and liver disease
- Severe Arthritis – see Jatinder's story in Part Four.
- Krohns Disease, Irritable Bowel and Colitis – see Dave Klein's story in Part Four.
- Hyperactivity, ADHD, behaviour issues – removing processed sugars, food additives and other stimulants, and instead supplying key minerals and vitamins for healthy brain function, reducing acidity and raising alkalinity etc.
- Candida – an all or high raw diet is often used to tackle candida, providing high quality nutrition whilst the foods that feed the candida imbalance are removed from the diet.
- Asthma, allergies and eczema – removing sources of irritation, reaction and tension, alkalising the system and providing good quality fats and oils to feed the skin.

Generally, the higher the percentage of raw food the greater the benefits. Or, the less you change from a normal diet, the less likely you are to see any real benefit. In essence, *corrupted biochemistry in foods of course creates corrupted biochemistry in the body*, so the smaller the proportion of corrupted biochemistry in the diet, the more the body can balance and rebuild its own robust inner biochemistry. For example, in effect cancer cells are corrupted cells, and thrive in a carbon dioxide rich environment, struggling to survive in an oxygen rich environment. Cooked food, stress and poor circulation create a carbon dioxide rich environment that is ideal for the growth of cancer cells. Raw food is oxygen rich. Well balanced raw food nutrition, combined with exercise, good breathing, and other health creating activities (see next section) creates an oxygen rich system giving the immune system the full support of a nutrient rich diet.

It's worth saying again: diet is usually an absolutely essential part of getting a sustainable solution, or significant improvement to chronic illness, disease or general ill-health – but it is not the only factor. Exercise and breathing, meditation, attitudes and mindset - many factors are part of the picture. So diet alone is not the 'cure' and should not be the only response.

THE *EAT MORE RAW* PATH AS A SPIRITUAL JOURNEY

It's worth covering this subject as it can be relevant and very helpful to some, although others may just want to skip on to the next section. If you're uncertain, then keep reading here.

Changing your diet and lifestyle is likely to bring many challenges, and present you with many choices about change in yourself, as well as how you live your life. Although many people will only see the physical dimensions of cleansing and nutritional changes, what is happening is that much is being re-arranged in your inner world if you follow this path. I have mentioned the emotional dimensions of this already - the reality is that the changes emerging through the re-arranging of your inner physical world usually will be a great journey of self-exploration, self-discovery and self-development in an emotional and spiritual sense as well. So if that is the kind of journey you want to take, or are already taking in life, then this is a good path to follow.

This aspect of the raw journey is often a great surprise and a great joy to many people. Looking inside yourself to what is going on in your whole being, and not just the physical body, can help you identify emotional blockages and overcome spiritual challenges. It's no accident that fasting is a widely used ancient practice along many spiritual paths, alongside eating simply and naturally, for lengthy periods of time.

Spending time in places in nature is often another part of this path – the wonderful book *Children of the Sun* indicates how this path was taken by many, including Herman Hesse for example, an author who strongly influenced a particular generation of people.[76]

Often the raw journey will bring people closer to nature simply because the food they are eating is more directly connected with nature. Remember, Mahatma Gandhi practiced simple living with a high raw diet for many years of his life, seeing this as an essential part of his path of integration between a spiritual and political life. So for some in the raw world, such as Dr Gabriel Cousens, Rev George Malkmus, Viktoras Kulvinskas and Nuria Aragon Castro (Sibila), the spiritual journey and the optimum nutrition journey are one journey.

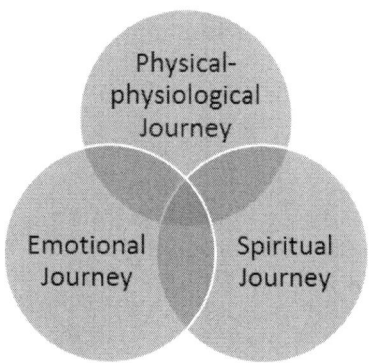

For many people on the eat more raw or real health path it is the spiritual path and awakening that accompanies it that is their primary interest, concern, challenge and joy. In this sense the lifestyle and the nutrition is merely a tool, like meditation or yoga, that can be used in the spiritual and personal development journey, and to great effect if practiced with deep integrity and clear intent.

---

[76] Gordon Kennedy, *Children of the Sun*, Nivaria Press (1998)

AN EASTERN SPIRITUAL PERSPECTIVE
The Tao of Health

The real focus of this book (or lack of it, if you get my drift) could be said to be 'the Tao of Health'. It's about a *Way* - possibly *The* way. That's what the Tao is – *The* Way - the indefinable way of the universe, which can be seen, 'tasted' and experienced in nature, and through nature.

This book then is about *the indefinable way of health*, which can be seen, 'tasted' and experienced in nature, and through nature. In this sense the 'eat more raw' thing is just a label. Don't attach to the label - see through and beyond it to the Way that is behind it - the Way that is drawn from, and emerges from, nature. The nature of health is seen in the plants, in the birds, in the soil, in the universal nature of things that can be sensed, experienced and lived. *The Way* that is out there in the world around us, and also in there, inside us waiting to be freed, by letting it simply be, flow and emerge. The Way of getting out of the way.

This *'Way of Health'* is philosophical, ethical and political, because it is a way of being in the world in daily life. It is the philosophy, ethics and politics of creating inner and outer health, in as many dimensions as possible – a powerful, change-making politics, that embodies the philosophy and ethics of pursuing the greater good of the one and the whole, together.

It could also be said to be religious - in the sense of seeking to know the divine, the ultimate, by experience - a state of true health can be seen as a divine gift, that is intended to be experienced. And the way of receiving that divine gift, is by following a path, as a self-directed spiritual way of life. It is a way that clearly emphasizes living in harmony with nature, and the Tao, which is both nature and much more than nature. It is a way of being on one's journey through life, following a "path" that is "principled"; that draws on the source of being, the source of health that is embodied in the Tao. In essence, the Tao is the place to go to *know* health. It is the force within and behind everything that exists, in its perfect state of being – and that inevitably is a state of what we can call 'health'.

As a Way of Health, in many cases this involves the 'action' of wu-wei - the action of non-action, getting out of the way, letting go of the obstacles in the way of health emerging, and of the Tao being expressed through whole health. This emphasizes simplicity, naturalness, spontaneity through connection with the Tao, compassion for yourself, your body and others, moderation particularly to avoid obsession, and a humility which allows that moderation to be. Humility is essential – real health does not exist in any form of self-obsession.

Although it is not essential or necessary, there can be a place for ritual, and for establishing familiar customs - for example in the preparation and enjoyment of natural, health giving food or a juice, or in its growing and harvesting. These are not set or fixed rituals or customs, and should certainly not become dogmatic, but they should be allowed to be if they have their place as a *meaningful* way of expressing the Tao through living a life of 'health' creation, which can be seen as an expression of the Tao. There can be a sacredness to them.

Whilst today, Taoism is still familiar in China and other parts of East and Southeast Asia, it is also known in the West - although I sense it is truly understood, or experienced, by few of us in the West. Taoism has been described as an "experience of the ultimate".[77] So being a 'successful' Taoist may lead to that experience – whereas calling yourself a Taoist may achieve nothing. In that sense *the Way* this book seeks to describe, and connect you with, is a Way that is in harmony with nature in both its inner and outer realms, that allows the health of inner and outer nature to be expressed, experienced and enjoyed. In this way, through its full and genuine expression, this represents an 'experience of the ultimate' – the ultimate possibility for health, of life, of the Tao, being lived in both the inner and outer realms of life.

This is *the un-nameable Way* this book seeks to connect you with.

A Confucian Approach to Health

From a Confucian perspective, an 'eat more raw' path is certainly an ethical and philosophical approach to living life according to certain principles – it is an ideology that is rooted in a certain ethical-sociopolitical perspective, that sees health as a natural rite for both people and nature, and that a greater good for all exists in the pursuit of this goal.

This way of life implies "the secular as sacred"[78]. It implies a practical order to life in a worldly-wise awareness of the rightness of health, with a respect to the divine nature of nature itself, and of health as a characteristic of nature. In its broader application it implies a deeply important role for the family and community, as the social units and social vehicles that bring about and sustain health, at any moment in time, and from generation to generation. This perspective embodies the belief that as human beings we are *'teachable, improvable, and perfectible through personal and communal endeavor especially self-cultivation and self-creation'*. It implies a focus on the cultivation of virtue and maintenance of ethics in order to bring about positive outcomes for the individual and society, which in turns implies an obligation to an altruistic way of life, the upholding of righteousness and the moral disposition to do 'good' as a creator of health. It implies a set of norms and principles that shape how we should act in everyday life to bring about the greater good of human and environmental health. It encourages an ability both to see and state clearly what is right and fair in the behaviors of others, and to see and state clearly what is wrong and unfair. As such it holds a certain level of passive or active contempt for those who fail to consider or uphold the right of health in others. In this sense it holds a more active contempt for those that through their way of life actively bring ill-health to others, but with no contempt for those that are ill.

A Buddhist Path to Health

From a Buddhist perspective, an eat more raw path is a "right way of living" that will free the 'Buddha of health' within, in the sense that, more than anything else, 'health' will *arise from an inner awakening*. This path can arise from adopting and consistently following certain beliefs and practices - or it can arise from instantaneous awakening.

---

[77] Meister, edited by Chad; Copan, Paul (2010). *The Routledge companion to philosophy religion* (1st paperback ed.). London: Routledge.

[78] A term used by philosopher Herbert Fingarette.

Try it, awaken now!

So the Dharma or 'path' involves sharing insights to help sentient beings (including the being that is Gaia) to end the suffering that arises from ill-health, sickness and dis-ease, by removing ignorance and craving for the things that generate ill-health, sickness and disease. The ultimate goal is the attainment of a sublime state of health, in every dimension of being, which can be achieved by practicing the Noble Eightfold Path to Health (which could also be called the Middle Way to Health)

The particular path to liberation from ill-health/suffering may vary, although a good deal is available to help you in this way of life, especially those practices that clearly generate health – cleansing, rebuilding and then maintaining vibrant health. From this perspective, there is no deity involved in health - it is a worldly thing. The foundations of this path are the 'triple gem' of:

- the 'Buddha of Health' – connection with an 'enlightened' or aware state of 'whole health';
- the pursuit of a 'Buddhist Way of Health' and its teachings;
- the community or culture of health creation.

Taking "refuge in the triple gem" represents a commitment to being on this path. Other practices may include adopting particular ethical principles, being part of a wider community that lives and teaches this life, renouncing conventional unhealthy living, cultivation of higher wisdom and discernment in pursuit of this path, study of the 'scriptures' of natural health creation, and practices as devotions to health creation.

The Samsara of Ill-Health: Going further into this Buddhist approach to health creation for people and planet, it is a path that seeks to release us from the samsara of the continual repetitive cycle of ill-ness that arises from people grasping and fixating on the experiences of the modern, ways of life that 'naturally' generate illness and suffering. Specifically, this path can be a way of generating a very real *rebirth* in physical realm or a psychological state, by adopting this way of life in a dedicated and committed way. It recognizes that without this we will continue to live in a state of ignorance, suffering, anxiety and dissatisfaction. From this perspective, liberation from 'the samsara of ill-health' is possible by following this path.

Karma: This path is rooted in an understanding of the 'Karmic' cycle which drives the creation of either ill-ness or health - both being natural 'karmic' outcomes of the thinking and actions expressed in our way of life. Our deeds or actions produce "seeds" in the mind and body which come to fruition in this life. The avoidance of unwholesome actions and the cultivation of positive actions are thus central to an "ethical conduct" which seeks to generate whole health. This karma of health is directly linked to the actions of body, speech or mind that spring from our mental intent in these matters, and which bring about a natural consequence, fruit or result in life.

Rebirth: We can bring about a fundamental *Rebirth* within our life – this arises from a fundamental transformation in our mind, body and spirit, as a result of in-life karmic forces. It arises from initiating processes whereby we are able to release ourselves from a repeating cycle. We have no permanent self, either as a 'whole being' or as a body, and ultimately there is no self that is independent from the rest of the universe, society and the environment. There is only fundamental inter-dependence, and Rebirth in this sense is part of the continuation of a dynamic, ever-changing process of "dependent arising" (of people and planet) shaped by the laws of cause and effect.

The Four Noble Truths of Health: The Four Noble Truths can provide a conceptual framework for a Buddhist pursuit of whole health. As the Four Noble Truths explain a) the nature of *dukkha* (suffering, anxiety, unsatisfactoriness), b) its causes, and c) how it can be overcome, they can be used as a fundamental framework to guide our understanding of health.

The four noble truths in this health-creating context are:

1. The truth of ill-health as a dimension of *dukkha* (suffering, anxiety, dis-ease)
2. The truth of the origin of ill-health
3. The truth of the cessation of ill-health
4. The truth of the path leading to the cessation of ill-health

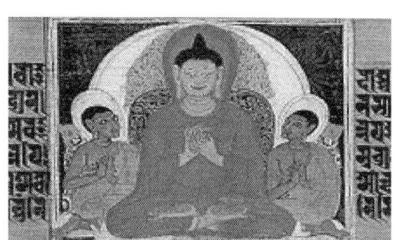
Buddha teaching the Four Noble Truths

The first truth explains the nature of what is commonly translated as "suffering", "anxiety", "unsatisfactoriness", "unease", etc., which relate to the multiple dimensions ill-health and dis-ease. This does not mean that Dukkha should be translated to mean ill-health or dis-ease. However, it can be seen as containing the following three aspects:

- The obvious suffering of physical and mental illness, unhealthy ageing and dying.
- The anxiety or stress of trying to seek health within a culture of ill-health.
- A subtle dissatisfaction arising from being without an inner core of natural health.

The second truth is that the origin of ill-health and dis-ease can be known and understood as arising from craving and attachment to those things that naturally create ill-health, which in turn arises from ignorance. Thus on a deeper level, *the root cause of ill-ness and dis-ease is ignorance of the true nature of health.*

The third noble truth is that a complete cessation of ill-health is possible.
The fourth noble truth identifies that there is a path to achieve this.

The Middle Way

An important guiding principle of this Buddhist approach to health creation is that of the Middle Way, which has several components:

1. The practice of non-extremism: a path of moderation away from the extremes of self-indulgence, self-mortification and self-obsession;
2. The middle ground between certain metaphysical perspectives, and ways of being, such as attachment or non-attachment to anyone perspective;
3. A state of awareness where it is continuously apparent that all dualities, paradoxes and polarization expressed by humanity in the world result from delusions;
4. A sense of peaceful emptiness, which avoids the polarities of permanence and nihilism, existence and nothingness.

The Noble Eightfold Path to Health

From a Buddhist approach, the path to health creation consists of pursuing a set of eight interconnected ways of being, that when progressed together, lead to the creation of health, and the cessation of illness, dis-ease and suffering. Thus, the path is about embodying in life and daily activities a connected, self-supporting web of factors, to naturally manifest health. These are not stages of health, they are significant dimensions of behavior that define a complete way of being in the world, and can be seen as covering three areas, as shown below.

Division	Eightfold factor	Description
Wisdom	1. Right view	Viewing the reality of health as it is, not just as it appears to be
	2. Right intention	Intention of creating health, including renunciation and freedom from that which creates ill-health, and harmlessness
Ethical conduct	3. Right speech	Speaking in a truthful, health-creating and non-hurtful way
	4. Right action	Action that contributes to whole health, and that is non-harmful
	5. Right livelihood	A livelihood that actively creates or contributes to whole health, as much or more than a non-harmful livelihood
Concentration	6. Right effort	Making an effort to improve health in oneself and the world
	7. Right mindfulness	Awareness to see things for what they are with clear consciousness; being aware of the present reality within oneself, without any craving or aversion
	8. Right concentration	Correct meditation or concentration, as a contribution to the on-going process of creating whole health

---------------------- o ----------------------

These philosophical yet practical approaches to life are vitally important for the adoption, development and strengthening of an entirely healthy relationship between oneself, society and the Earth as a whole, because they prevent the kind of self-obsessed approach to health that can be common in the 'me-oriented' western consumer culture. In this sense these 'ways of being in the world' take us closer to a path that, in its healthiest state, integrates into one a conscious socially, politically and spiritually 'revolutionary' path, which places love for people, nature and creation as the ultimate path to personal, social and spiritual fulfillment.

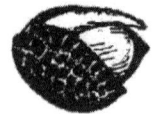

SPROUTED HEMP SEED - FANTASTIC NUTRITION!

EAT MORE RAW PARENTING – BEFORE AND AFTER BIRTH

CHILDREN IN GENERAL

Some active and otherwise healthy children seem to have a constantly running nose or skin problems - this is often the natural result of that child's immune system being active and healthy, ridding itself of the mucus and toxins that come into its body through a typical western diet. Paradoxically, many children on the worst diets or who are well over-weight are often not detoxing and don't get such bad colds because their body has too much to cope with already in 'just surviving' mode. This is quite obviously not because they are healthier.

Depending on the family circumstances, it may or may not be easy to help children establish a *truly healthy* diet or lifestyle, however a lot can be done to establish a *healthier* diet and lifestyle. Fortunately there are now plenty of books, magazines and networks available to help. The main issue is that normally the child wants to copy the parent - well, younger children tend to, clearly it's not necessarily the same with teenagers! Teenagers want to copy idols and role models. Whatever the age of the children, if the parent is happy and relaxed during any cleansing, and happy eating more raw foods, the child will be much more likely to be too.

When you step back and look from a natural health perspective, many of the ideas and practices around childbirth that our culture accepts as 'normal' start to look rather weird and surreal. From a natural health and natural parenting perspective it is bizarre that pregnancy and childbirth is more or less treated as a medical condition in the west, with many mothers-to-be racked with fear of childbirth rather than confidence. This was particularly apparent to me over the months during which I was preparing to become a father for the first time – and fortunately my partner at the time was not someone who bought into that fear, trusting in nature and her womanhood. Nature has taken millions of years to evolve and develop the ideal conditions for childbirth and pregnancy - once this is realised it's possible for these fears to reduce, and for confidence to emerge in its place, which is of course healthy for the fetus / baby.

The benefits of healthy nutrition for children, before and after birth, cannot be overstressed. It is now widely accepted that healthy nutrition at this stage makes a difference through our whole life. Information sources and books to help parents and children with more naturally healthy and enjoyable lifestyles are growing in number - including books and websites for those wanting to eat more raw and to 'transition' kids and family to a healthy diet and lifestyle, with many excellent resources listed in the appendices section of this book.

There are many issues that parents meet when transitioning a family to a healthier lifestyle - food is only one – and many people have now gone through this process. A great number of parents find that their children actually love eating more raw foods (though some will not - it varies from child to child). Generally, the earlier they start eating more raw the better. There can be challenges if kids have already got into processed or junk foods, but you can be confident that there is plenty of good experience, guidance and support now available to you, and that it often turns out to be a wonderful and positive experience for both children and parents alike.

Working on the second edition of this book, as a parent I'm now a few years down the line (as of 2015, my son is 8). The following is distilled primarily from the experience of others, alongside my observations of those who are most successful, and from of my own experience:

- The parent(s)'s state of mind is the most important thing: younger kids copy parents, teenagers need freedom and mentors, or 'idols'. If you are at ease with the changes and with your lifestyle, excited and enthusiastic about them, then usually the children will be too (particularly younger children). It's no help to your child if you become fearful or paranoid about 'bad food'. Focus on your own healthy mental attitude and emotions rather than on the food so that the kids can *enjoy* a more naturally healthy way of living. Be creative, make it a game and an adventure, and also make sure it is something that gives them (and you) a sense of security, confidence and love.
- Be aware that kids often love savoury foods, sometimes more than sweet foods – they often love to eat cucumber for example, so just make it easy for them to eat plenty of any raw fruit or veg they particularly enjoy. As well as cucumber, my son also loves sweet (bell) peppers, 'carrot cars' and carrot 'spaghetti', dehydrated crackers, rocket, wild garlic and chives – these tastes have evolved over time, as he has grown and had the freedom to try for himself.
- When they are ready, giving babies and toddlers a bowl to pick from with two or three of the following is great – blueberries, banana or pear slices, pieces of avocado, soaked goji berries, raspberries, and so on.
- When pregnant and breast feeding, make sure you have/mum has a fresh juice (e.g. apple and carrot) at least every morning to start the day - often with high quality DHA (e.g. NuTru's OmegaZen) and mineral supplements, such as those supplied by Marine Minerals - and when the little one is ready, prepare them a small glass at the same time. Letting them sip from mum's glass helps them get going on this. Keeping a fresh juice going every day for kids of all ages is great, and at a certain point they'll want to be able to make them themselves.
- Colourful and interesting foods, as well as delicious foods, can help a lot. There is now a fantastic range of recipes that are ideal for children – again see the resources section.
- Children detox more directly, and most kids on a 'normal' diet get horrible colds and mucus anyway, but usually they finish as quickly as they start. By improving their diet, the detox process will clear mucus out, which will not feel any different to a bad cold to the child, and leave them clearer, depending on the degree and type of raw foods they eat, and what else they eat. If they have been on sugary foods, foods with additives or junk food they may get some bad headaches and be sensitive or grumpy for a day or two. If they eat 50% raw and 50% junk they will be very 'snotty'; if they eat 50% raw or more, and the rest is mainly carefully selected cooked organic wholefoods they will normally be in pretty good shape, provided they are on low / zero dairy or wheat, which are two big mucus producers.
- There are challenges for one parent if the other is not supportive of the healthier diet, especially if it seems extreme. In these situations it is better to be clear that you just want the child to eat more healthily, with plenty of fruit and raw vegetables, and to cut out junk foods. It may well make things *more* difficult if you talk or think about 'going raw', or are unwilling to look at a middle-ground or a degree of compromise. Whatever the level of raw foods, *you can usually make sure your child is getting a healthier nutritional start than you did*. A compromise can be to mix very healthy foods with typical staples, such as bananas mashed with flax/omega oils, mixed with organic porridge (cooled a bit), with oat-milk and a few gojis, blueberries and raisins sprinkled on top. Any parent, whatever their own diet, can offer this kind of healthier option as a start to their child, both for the day and for life.

- Inventing your own recipes with the kids is great fun for all involved, and is much easier than cooked recipes. As an example: banana blended with half an orange, raisins, pumpkin seeds, omega oil, flax seeds, goji berries, spring water and a bit of this and that in my home it's known as 'Dada porridge', and provides a nutritious breakfast that my son really enjoys especially with some goji's, blueberries or date. Also you can be confident with raw 'sweets'/puddings, knowing they are healthy for your children, giving them the quality nutrition they need – rather than being really damaging to their teeth, creating hyperactivity or being potentially fattening and addictive (there are now quite a number of healthy raw / mainly raw snack bars e.g. Yaoh, Raw chocolate bars, etc).
- Dehydrators for making raw crackers and a good blender for making a range of raw puddings can be very useful – my son enjoys both the making and the eating.
- With salads, get the kids involved in growing the salads as well as making them. They can learn and be excited by this in itself, they will also make the direct connection with the food, and will be much more excited about eating salads when they have grown or helped to grow them themselves. Often kids (like my son) like crunchy chunks of carrot, cucumber and pepper – rather than green leaves. Let them have what they enjoy, and be prepared to let them find the greens they like. Green juices or greens blended with seed milks (and then strained) are an option - for some children the fact that a green juice looks 'weird' is enough to grab their interest, and test their courage to experiment and have a go. Others will just say 'yuk!'.

Generally, you can use the whole process of change as an education process, helping the kids to understand where their food comes from geographically (and economically) and from what types of plants, how it is grown, and how it makes the body naturally healthy. *The fact that they will be growing up knowing that there are different possibilities to a conventional diet is something that will stay with them for the rest of their life – this is really important. The fact that they make a direct link between food and health will always be with them*, and in 20 years when they are adults and the world has moved on it may be much easier to make very healthy choices than it is today.

PREGNANT AND BREAST FEEDING MUMS

Diet pre-conception, during pregnancy and in the early years is increasingly recognized as *hugely important* for the whole of a person's life. Key nutrients for you/mums at this stage are essential for proper fetal development – and can be provided either within foods (including juices or smoothies) or with high quality nutritional supplements. Some of the key ones are:

1. B12 – vital for healthy brain/neurological development; essential for any pregnant or breast feeding mothers, particularly vegans.
2. Zinc – especially ionic zinc;
3. Flax/linseed or hemp oil (keep refrigerated) - 1 desert-spoon/day with other foods;
4. Supplement of multiple trace minerals – an excellent source is www.marineminerals.com, e.g. their Lightening Tablets;
5. DHA supplement – e.g. O-Mega-Zen by NuTru, available from various US sources including Vegan Essentials and from www.detoxyourworld.com in the UK;
6. Barley greens / food state greens powder e.g. E3Live and others (look particularly for field grown or rock re-mineralised, and/or wild-crafted greens); AND / OR

7. Green juices, green seed milks, etc – nettles and spinach are great, as is kale – e.g. when juicing combine the green leaves with a little lemon, some apple and carrot, or other combinations; with milks blend nettles with hemp seed and spring water, and then strain for an amazing source of nutrition – a dash of flax oil can be added, and a Marine Minerals *Lightening Tablet* or two; highly recommended!

If you include all or most of the above in a pre-conception, pregnancy and/or breast-feeding diet, or an early years diet, you will be providing excellent nutrition to yourself and your child. The appendices section lists more fully a range of sources for high quality supplements and super foods, as well as a great range of recipes.

During pregnancy do not over-do it, and detox too heavily. Morning sickness is a detoxification process, which can be intense, but which is manageable for the body's systems. Do not over-stretch it. As a minimum during and after any pregnancy, and whilst breast feeding, high quality building foods are key, and I would highly recommend the simple combination of:

- a fresh juice to start *every* morning with a DHA capsule (e.g. O-Mega-Zen from NuTru) and several Marine Minerals *Lightning tablets* or a few drops of their *Liquid Trace Minerals* (or similar) added to the juice.
- An ideal afternoon/evening addition is a green juice or greens/seed milk combination e.g. nettles and hemp/sunflower, plus some flax oil, blended together and strained.

The brain, neurological system and organs are all significantly built of fats, so they all need high quality fats for their building process during infancy, childhood and in pregnancy. At the same time vitamins and minerals are essential catalysts in the metabolizing of nutrients, so these are also needed for healthy nutrition for the child and pregnant mother. Furthermore, Tony Wright's work suggests a key role for the flavonoids associated with colour in fruits and vegetables in the process of gene transcription. This suggests that regular home-made fresh raw smoothies and puddings made with fruit and soaked seeds, plus omega oils and some berries (e.g. goji, blueberry, etc), with some high quality mineral supplements are a darned good idea for children and pregnant and breast feeding mums.

Given the nature of our culture, much of the natural health and raw food movements have been very 'me' focused. Now the emerging maturity within some parts of the raw food movement will increasingly recognize that *mother and child health is fundamental to the health of the next generations*. Following some early pioneers, when they are considering becoming mothers, more women within the movement are realizing that a different kind of approach to diet and nutrition is needed pre-pregnancy, during pregnancy, during extended breast feeding well beyond 1 year, and throughout infancy and childhood. Deeper research and understanding will develop by mothers working together in this area. Optimum biochemistry/nutrition for the health and resilience of the human reproductive system in its broadest sense is perhaps more important than anything. Time will tell.

The books on raw parenting listed in the appendices give a great deal of advice based on genuine personal experiences as well as a wide range of excellent recipes designed to excite the taste and meet the nutritional needs of children. Rather than attempting to address all the issues here, I recommend that parents explore this themselves and take advantage of the books and contacts listed in the appendices so that they can learn from experienced experts.

F.A.Q's About The Practicalities of Eating More Raw

FAQ1 - How do I go to roughly 50% raw, 50% cooked? How is this best achieved? What foods should I eat and when?

Firstly, get off fried foods, junk foods and processed foods, completely, as soon as you can – say over 2 weeks. To start moving towards 50% raw, have fresh fruit for breakfast and snack on fruit during the morning if necessary. For very active people really filling up on fruit is fine for breakfast, with some fresh+dried fruit top-ups along the way later. Fruit-only mornings is the best first step and will soon bring more energy and clarity, after the early cleansing in the first few days, or first week or so. In these early days or weeks, and during any more intense cleansing phases that follow when the body is ready, you will feel weary, so remember to rest and refer to the detox and cleansing sections earlier in the book.

In addition to the fruit-only mornings: a) ideally have one type of ripe fresh fruit at least 30 minutes before other meals (because ripe fruit digests quickly), and/or b) have a salad of raw vegetables as the first part of every main meal, and at least a salad of raw vegetables and greens as part of every main meal – see the Recipes appendix for numerous examples of the types of 'salads' I'm talking about here. These should not be boring old lettuce, cucumber, tomato and onion salads unless you particularly like that!

To get to 50% raw or more fairly easily, work with a selection of the raw recipes in this book and others, and get to know what you like most. Get comfortable and confident with about 10 or 15 different basic salad ingredients, with some particular favourites – you can change the mixes, proportions and combinations of these, with a few exotic ingredients if you like and then you'll find that every salad tastes deliciously different. And if you do these things then I'll bet you'll find that you're less bored than with your previous diet! Ideally, aim to make at least two meals a day raw, or one raw meal and two half-raw, with raw snacks (e.g. fruit) in between.

If you can fit in some kind of cleanse early on, this will help make the 50:50 target easier – and take time off for that if you're working. A good programme of exercise will help too.

In summary 50% raw is relatively easily achieved if you stick at it for a month at least (from one full moon to the next works well), especially by working with the following:

100% raw / all or mainly fruit mornings;   Raw snacks between meals;
Minimum 50%+ raw lunch;   A good-sized, tasty salad with every evening meal;
Fruit before evening meal;   Raw puddings, raw sweets and raw treats;

And if you don't get to 50% raw, be happy with where you've got to, keep it up, and try again for the 50% target in a month or two

FAQ2 - Will the food be satisfying enough?

The simple answer is 'yes'... when you learn what satisfies you. The initial transition to an eat more raw lifestyle is when you may worry about being satisfied. Seed/nut dips and patés are all very satisfying. Dried fruit, nuts and seeds, and the more fatty raw foods are good fillers too. An Israeli family I met in Spain, with four boys, found that eating fruit before a main salad meal lead to satisfaction for them. While, a carpenter, working long days in London, found that a large fruit salad for breakfast with plenty of bananas and some tahini kept him satisfied right through the day, until he got back home for an evening salad.

Many people (particularly hard working, heavy eating men) find that fairly soon (e.g. 3 weeks) after switching to eating more raw they are *more* satisfied, *eating less* - because the food they are eating has a lot more nutrition in it and better combinations make it easy to digest. So they can get more nutrition, eating less. This is also particularly noticeable if you switch to eating all or mainly organic foods and if you chew your food properly.

For a filling breakfast alternative to only fruit, blend together bananas or other fruit with pumpkin seed, sunflower seed and flax seed (ideally soaked overnight), with raisins or dates, some omega / flax oil, and possibly other ingredients like goji berries, with a little water added.

Four relatively harmless bulk cooked foods are potatoes (best steamed or boiled), oats and millet, or quinoa. These foods require relatively little processing, are whole foods, and need relatively little energy to cook. Organic rolled oats are acidifying but can be used in moderation if soaked in water and uncooked. Millet requires little processing and can be cooked just by bringing to the boil for a few minutes and then turning the heat off and leaving it for 5 to 10 minutes – importantly Millet is also the only alkaline grain.

These were foods that I ate as basic fillers when I was transitioning to raw foods, and later in a mainly raw diet.[79] If you substitute these and other foods for wheat pasta / bread, meat and dairy, even if you don't eat much more raw food you will be doing yourself and the planet a great deal of good. Along with steamed vegetables they are relatively harmless cooked food fillers. And remember not to combine badly, particularly if you are still eating cooked starches.

FAQ3 - WHAT IS A TYPICAL DIET FOR A WEEK?

A typical diet for a week? Again, that's a good question - but whose typical diet do you mean? And what time of the year? Where are they on their health journey, and what's going on in their typical week? For example, do most people eat the same in the depths of winter as they do in the summer? What climate and culture are they in? Do they grow some of their own food? Are they regular snackers or are they only main meal eaters? Do they buy from an organic veggie box scheme, a local market or do they buy mail-order or from a supermarket?

Whilst it's a good question, there is of course no such thing as a typical person or a typical week – so there's no off-the-shelf, out-of-the-packet answer. For that reason I'm not giving you a general menu or meal plan here that might not suit your character, your tastes and your needs - instead I'm giving you plenty of options and helpful pointers in the right direction. I want you to know that you can explore a variety of options, and that by experiment *you will find out what suits you*.

But I also have some very helpful hints that add to the previous two FAQ answers:

---

[79] I don't include rice because it often involves a lot of food miles and commercial rice growing (like cattle farming) releases a lot of methane into the atmosphere - a greenhouse gas 20 times more powerful than CO_2, and therefore a significant contributor to climate change.

- Juices and smoothies are simple and delicious – they work really well for a lot of people, so find out if they work for you, and try a few different types.
- Start by buying more of a variety of fruit and veg than you normally do – then pick what you fancy for breakfast, lunch and supper, perhaps with a raw humus or seed'n'veg paté for supper, or an avocado dish with whatever salad you choose to create for lunch, and a decent fruit/raw breakfast. And make sure there's plenty of foods you really enjoy in there of course.
- Get yourself a good fruit bowl, if you don't have one, and keep it well stocked. And get yourself a beautiful salad bowl that's a pleasure to use.
- Make sure your week's food supply includes a number of options for raw fats, sugars and proteins but remember that *greens* are the best source for minerals and for building proteins, so don't overdo the nuts and seeds.
- Most people do well with fruit/raw breakfasts and morning snacks, with some preferring fruit lunches with a salad in the evening. Others like main salads for lunch and fruit in the evening, and some a salad for both lunch and supper. I started with fruit in the morning and salads for lunch and supper. At 4 to 6 months I naturally shifted to a fruit lunch too, with a salad just in the evening. This has been my basic pattern since about 1995, with a few variations here and there, depending on how I feel at the time. Find the pattern that works for you.
- Your diet is likely to change over time. Your body will want to cleanse early on - you can help it with more juices, with intensive juicing over a weekend for example. Essentially, if you keep at it over several months or ideally at least a year, and combine the improved nutrition coming in with gradual cleansing and good exercise to keep the metabolism working well, then your eat more raw lifestyle will become increasingly stable, balanced and easy over time.

FAQ4 - WHAT DO I DO ABOUT SOURCING ALL THE INGREDIENTS...?

As far as sourcing goes, you have several choices.

1) Firstly, I do <u>not</u> recommend buying everything from your local supermarket – as they sell what suits them (which to me is mostly junk), in terms of profits, marketing and stock management. Mostly they sell highly processed foods in plastic packaging, cans, cartons, boxes and bottles – whilst the fresh food they sell is often not ripe or the best quality in terms of its nutritional value even if it looks spotless and shiny. Supermarkets tend to destroy local food markets and supply networks, and often treat their suppliers very harshly. They encourage you to drive, and the vast, vast majority of the stuff they sell as 'food' is actively creating or sustaining chronic illness much more than it is creating health. To me, if you buy from supermarkets you are supporting the profits of those who sell more foods that tend to create chronic illness, rather than health. That's my little supermarket rant done with![80] It's up to you whether you listen to my rant of course.

2) If you prefer it fresh and local, there are normally people out there to do that too. Local organic farm shops, organic veggie box schemes and wholefood stores are your greatest

---

[80] See the acclaimed book by Joanna Blythman, *Shopped! The Shocking Truth About UK Supermarkets*, Harper Perennial (2005) – a great expose of the true nature and effects of our supermarket culture.

resources - along with your garden, backyard, window boxes or allotment. Increasingly raw super foods like Goji berries, as well as raw snack bars and raw chocolate bars, are available in regular whole food stores – it's so much easier now than it was ten or even five years ago! (You can even grow Goji's in much of the UK). Then there can be farmer's markets, regular markets and local wholesalers, who often have ripe fruit and veg at really good prices. Really have a go at growing at least some of your own greens if you can – it makes a big difference.

3)   If you like phone/internet mail order and bulk buying then there's now plenty of choice for very high quality foods, made easy for you (e.g. getting organic seeds, dried fruit and nuts from wholefood suppliers such as Suma, Infinity, etc in the UK). One approach (if you can afford it) is to buy lots of raw superfoods and supplements from organisations such as Funky Raw or Detox Trading (my preferred suppliers, with a sensible range and good prices), Detox Your World, Raw Living or the Fresh Network, or Organics Direct in Britain by email / mail order, or from Nature's First Law or other raw suppliers in the US. It is great that these options are available, and buying key foods is great. However, occasionally an unhealthy obsession with these products can set in – if taken too far it is generally high on 'food miles' (and therefore CO_2 emissions), expensive, involves a lot of packaging and can lead people to feel dependent on a lot of "raw superfoods" (and the companies that supply them) - which they are not. I didn't buy *any* of these things for more than 10 years on my raw path, and did fine without them, and was in fact at my healthiest because I was getting a vibrant variety of fresh greens every day as my raw superfoods.

4)   If you like a bit of both of 2) and 3) above then go for that. This tends to be my preference, mainly buying local and bulk wholefoods, with a bit of the specialist raw supplies added in (particularly for the family).

FAQ5 - How do you stop a raw diet/lifestyle becoming boring?

Well, that's a good question isn't it? And my immediate answer is: how do you stop a cooked food diet/lifestyle becoming boring?! It's easy, if you make your food interesting and enjoyable, which is as simple with raw foods as with cooked. There's a vast array of recipes, combinations, super simple or complex 'cordon raw' approaches that you can try. Raw foods are definitely no more boring than cooked foods and have at least as many opportunities for creativity and awesome, amazing flavour-full experiences. In fact, once they're eating more raw, many people find they can taste 'a lot more and a lot better' – so they enjoy their food more. This is because the taste system becomes cleansed and the tastes of raw foods are really fresh and alive.

It's easy to experiment with raw foods and it's difficult to make raw disasters (while cooked disasters are easy to achieve!). There are plenty of subtle or spicy flavours to play with, and a host of exciting food combinations to explore. On the fruit side you can try deliciously simple mixes like orange or grapefruit and avocado, apple and avocado, or banana and avocado. On the salad or main meal side try a raw curry, carrot and ginger, or believe it or not, finely chopped leek and grated parsnip with a little olive oil, lemon juice and a dash of tamari is delicious. Using different seaweeds in salads, raw vegan 'sushi'/nori rolls and other dishes provides yet another dimension to taste experiments.

With any type of food often it is the texture as much as the flavour that people get bored by, so it's important to experience variety in terms of the nutrition, flavours, textures and the look of the food. Personally I'm not really into recipes – I like to just create what I feel like at the time, and over the years I've had consistently good results like this. However, there's a good selection of recipes included in the appendices section of this book to help you – donated by people who have been through the transition experience themselves, and their tried and tested delicious offerings are carefully selected to aid that process.

A trick to help you from conventional 'haute cuisine' is that if the following five flavours are included to some extent in a meal it is very likely to be satisfying to the tastebuds:

- Sweet   Salty   Sharp/Sour   Spicy/Pungent   Bitter.

Try it out a few times and you'll taste the difference!

FAQ6 - WHAT'S THE IDEAL RAW DIET?

There is no ideal, off-the-shelf raw diet that suits everyone. However, there are a wide range of *opinions* on an ideal raw diet. So remember, just because people are forthright or their diet is right for them, it doesn't mean it's right for others.

Many factors influence what's best for you at any one time – state of health, personality, age, climate, mental attitudes and emotional state, stage in the cleansing / transition process, dietary history, relationships and so on - all these factors change over time. I recommend trying a variety of balances in your diet, and different cleansing approaches, over a period of time, because what suits you at the start of the path (more balanced towards cleansing or healing) may change later (more sustaining, or rebuilding) as more stable levels of health are gained.

In fact the idea of an ideal raw diet, or of an ideal raw fooder, often does more harm than good. It sets many people up to fail, often leading to feelings of guilt, shame or failure because of "slippage", and not being 'perfect'. So be realistic and give yourself time and flexibility. Some people can stay very focused, or just love their new diet and lifestyle, and for them the raw ideal can be something they can pursue in a balanced way. So I am not saying it's not possible. Also, it can be much easier if you are in a very supportive environment for a lengthy period of time. But for most, if you are realistic you will set yourself up to be successful by not falling into the trap of thinking there's a single ideal raw diet and there's something wrong with you if you fail to maintain it - instead keep taking significant steady, practical and achievable steps towards the goal of improved health and well-being, with roughly 50%+ raw as an 'ideal' initial target.

FAQ7 - WHAT EXTRA EQUIPMENT WOULD I NEED? IS A JUICER ESSENTIAL?

The only things that are essential are a knife, a bowl and a chopping board... and even they are optional for some! A juicer can be an excellent investment to speed the cleansing process, but is not essential. Centrifugal juicers are cheaper, less efficient but a great start – I had one that I used a lot and worked well for about 10 years. Juicers like GreenPower or Champion juicers (masticating juicers) are more expensive, but much more sturdy and efficient at getting the juice out – and are more multi-functional e.g. for making raw pate, or raw chocolate. Hand-juicers can be good for green juices. Be careful with the expensive juicers – GreenPower market themselves as the best juicers in the world, which they may be for greens and for their multi-functionality - in my experience a Champion is better if you're mainly juicing fruit and root vegetables like carrots. Choose according to what juices you will make, and other processing needs you have.

Food processors are used by many people – and hand processors (mincers, seed grinder, pestle and mortar), can be as good as electric ones, are more ecological, and are great for seed patés, raw cakes and raw curries. The Vitamix is the queen of the blenders / processors, and whilst expensive, will last much longer than cheaper models and is more versatile. And the Nutribullet makes life very simple for high quality smoothies.

Dehydrators are considered essential by some. For some they are great, particularly for producing raw versions of some standard cooked dishes, and for catering for kids. But for others, they are simply not necessary. It's up to your tastes, what you like to do in terms of food preparation, and whether you like a lot of kitchen gadgets, or prefer simplicity. And remember, if you're in a warm or hot climate (including summer in temperate climates) you can easily use the sun as a dehydrator. For most of my raw path I have not used a dehydrator – when I use one now it is mainly for variety, friends/guests or my son.

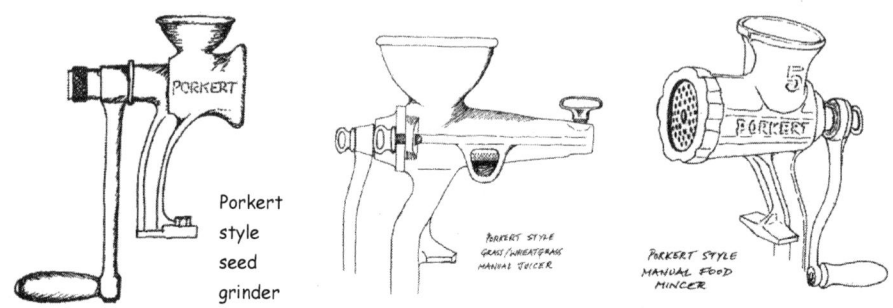

Porkert style seed grinder

PORKERT STYLE GRASS/WHEATGRASS MANUAL JUICER

PORKERT STYLE MANUAL FOOD MINCER

If you feel that the high quality equipment is very expensive, then consider comparing it to the cost of health care and being sick – it tends to look cheap in comparison. Or look at the equipment's cost per day divided over five years. You don't actually need any of these things – but for many they do really help. Remember, some of the greatest, most amazing salads and other dishes are easily produced by hand. You don't have to switch from a cooker, freezer or microwave dependency to a blender, juicer and dehydrator dependency – simplicity is safe, enjoyable and delicious! The simplest and most affordable implements to use, clean and maintain are quite simply the simplest implements – good knives, a great chopping board and beautiful bowls. And generally the fresher your food and the more you grow your own the less you will bother about equipment and gadgets, because as a rule the freshest food is always the tastiest and the best.

FAQ8 - WHAT ARE THE BEST THINGS TO SPROUT?

Among the best and simplest things to sprout are green lentils and chickpeas. Sunflower seeds are excellent if you have a good quality supply (poor quality seeds will rot quite quickly once soaked). Quinoa, aduki beans, black-eyed beans and alfalfa are also excellent. You'll find that different sprouts have different characters and that you can use them in different ways in a meal. For example, alfalfa and quinoa are great mixed in with greens, or other salad elements, with chickpeas being great to use in a raw humous as a satisfying, staple part of the salad.

Many people love mung beans (the 'bean sprouts' most often available in shops). Again you need a good supply, because if they don't all sprout they can create quite a crunch for the teeth. Green or puy lentils are simple, reliable and taste great (my favorite). Radish, mustard and fenugreek are great for something with more zap to it!

Sprouts provide really high quality organic nutrition *at a very, very low cost* – so they are fantastic for individuals and families on a low budget, including students. Getting a sprouting system going can also be fun. Sprouts are a very useful but not essential raw food - a well-designed diet can provide all your nutritional needs without them.

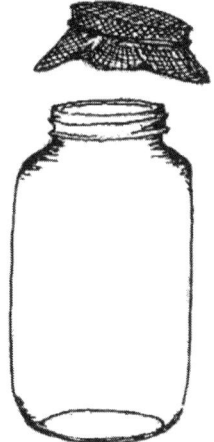

Sprouting Jar, with cloth or mesh top

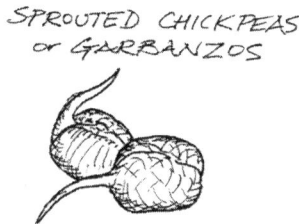

SPROUTED CHICKPEAS or GARBANZOS

The 'living foods' school of raw foodists promote sprouts - from that school Dr Brian Clements of Hippocrates Health Institute is one of the most respected of all raw food educators. Meanwhile the natural hygienists do not see them as a natural food for us – except in limited quantities of sprouted greens (e.g. the green shoots of sprouted sunflower seeds, which are delicious). Again, balance seems the best approach, and if sprouts work for you then great. If they don't, then don't worry, just make sure you are getting the nutrients they can provide in other ways.

The basics of sprouting are: soak the seeds / pulses overnight, no longer - small seeds such as alfalfa just need 4 to 6 hours - then drain, and rinse once or twice a day – they will normally be ready between 2 and 4 days. There are some excellent and cheap books on sprouting available from the main raw/living foods networks, such as Edward Kearney's *The Sprouting Handbook* and Sally Holloway's simple, affordable *Sprouting in the UK* (see Appendices for details).

FAQ9 - WHAT DO YOU EAT WHEN YOU'RE OUT, OR VISITING FRIENDS OR FAMILY?

Personally, when I visit friends and family or go out to a restaurant I have a very simple and effective strategy – I politely tell people *what I do want*, rather than focusing on what I don't want. Generally, this works well.

I have found that often chefs enjoy the opportunity to prepare something different. I always emphasise 'just vegetables and fruit, please – nothing cooked thank you'. If there's nothing obvious, I simply ask for the avocado in place of the salmon or chicken when such salads are on the menu. 'A simple French dressing is fine, thank you' works well, and whatever is on the menu asking for a simple avocado salad is one of the best strategies – or for vegetarians these days a goats cheese salad is often available, and if not all raw then salad with new potatoes is simple. Some do not rise to the challenge, but in general I have enjoyed some great salads with this simple, clear request. And I sometimes have a couple of apples with me, in case I get the sad lettuce, cucumber, tomato and onion cliché salad!

With friends, I'm always happy to bring some food or ingredients along. Often I offer to prepare salad dishes or raw dips and pates with them, which they tend to enjoy (the preparation and the eating) as they are often keen to try something new, interesting and different. Obviously this depends on what your friends are like, and maybe I have particularly open and interested friends! Being clear about what I do eat (rather than what I do not eat) makes it really simple, and it seems that a raw vegetable salad is easily understandable by most people – more so than requesting a macrobiotic meal for example.

My wider family are accepting of my choices, and whilst at first I found it difficult at times to eat alongside their meat or fish and cooked veg meals (because of my defensiveness about what I was doing, in those early days), it's been as much a question of me adapting my perspective to them, as them adapting to my changes. They often enjoy sharing some of my exotic salad concoctions as part of their meals, and are always happy to buy in a few extra salad ingredients if I am visiting. Again, maybe I have been lucky with my family, friends and work colleagues. The main thing is: *be happy with what you are doing, and be clear that you enjoy it and feel better for it*, and not to apologise for it or feel you are being difficult – particularly if you offer to bring a salad or ingredients, or help in food preparation. Parents want to see their children healthy and happy, so whilst some parents may worry about your changes, if you are healthier and happier, over time they will see that.

When it comes to partners and/or children this can be a more complex issue. Differences in the family or relationship have their challenges, but most relationships have those, including all raw ones. So it's as much about how the challenge is responded to as the issue itself. Again, the main thing is to be clear in yourself and to do what feels right within the context of the relationship. If children are involved, then seek agreement between the parents on what constitutes a lovingly healthy diet, and use high quality food state supplements to guarantee key nutrients where possible, whether the diet is all or mainly raw or not. Virtually always you'll be able to find a balance that is healthier than it was before the 'eat more raw' option emerged in the family or relationship, and in time that balance will evolve and change in its own way. With children, be aware that if you work on it you can almost certainly give them a better start than you yourself may have had. If they aren't on what you feel is an ideal diet, health creating nutrition will at least become familiar to them, if you are eating it happily every day, which means they will at least see that as a choice or possibility in their own lives as they grow up, and throughout their life.

WHAT ARE THE BEST THINGS TO DRINK AND HOW IMPORTANT ARE THEY?

Generally, with the western diet most people are not sufficiently hydrated, so just drinking plenty of water will help improve health e.g. 2 litres per day. But also remember you're eating more foods with a lot more liquids in them when you eat more raw foods.

Like foods and fats, there are liquids that create health, and liquids that create illness. With an 'eat more raw diet' in some ways your foods become your drinks, especially with fruits, because generally they are liquid rich. In terms of liquids though, water is best and ideally spring water from a local spring – next best is filtered or bottled spring water (not gassed/carbonated).[81] Fresh juices (vegetable and fruit juices) are also excellent – meaning made by you or your host, and not bought juices (which are pasteurized) - though these are better than coffee or tea if you are making that change. Green super foods drinks are fine too. With tap water, it varies across countries - you should always use a filter jug or a fitted filter system – and it should be left to stand for some time to allow any chlorine to evaporate off. The world of water is a world of its own!

So if possible satisfy your thirst with water, fresh juice or fruit. Some people seem to drink more than others (and I'm in that category) – this may be more out of habit than biological necessity. Spring water with a little freshly squeezed lemon juice is a favourite in a hot climate. If you want a hot drink then herb teas are best, or plain hot water. For long periods I drank no hot drinks at all, but living back in the UK, and engaging in a more normal life (than when I was at Ecoforest) I happily drink herbal teas, and some other hot drinks. And, as far as other standard drinks in our society go let's start with coffee ... because from experience I know a fair bit about it, and it can be a tough bean to crack!

Coffee is a harsh drug to the system that will probably contribute to significant de-mineralisation of your body and eventually to a range of maladies if it is drunk in significant quantities over time (e.g. 2 or more cups / mugs per day for many years). If you are all or mainly raw, then the effects of coffee may be more severe. All this I know from my own experience of having been a coffee drinker for most of my life. If you want to give up coffee, using organic cocoa can be a useful transition or alternative with lower caffeine levels. The most useful alternative that I have found is green tea, which still has caffeine, but which is rich in antioxidants and certain bioflavonoids. Often sugar addiction is part and parcel of the coffee/caffeine addiction, so if you are struggling to give such things up be aware that it can be a tough one (for many but not all), so be compassionate with yourself and your addictions!

If you are drinking coffee a) cut-down, b) get off the instant stuff, as it's full of the dregs of the industry, in more senses than one, c) eat enough fats (avocado, raw nuts, seeds, oils, etc) as these seem to buffer the acidic effects of caffeine, and d) try a half-decaf, half-regular mix. Riding your coffee fueled bicycle, you won't avoid the caffeine pot hole, but you will make it smaller.

Tea is not much better than coffee, although shifting to weak black tea can be a pleasant change. Tea also contains significant caffeine, as well as tannin, which inhibits digestion. Like

---

[81] For conscious consumers, I suggest you look on the bottle to avoid the numerous Nestle, Danone or Coca Cola owned water companies, if you can find alternatives.

coffee, if you are used to drinking a lot of tea either give it up completely if you can, or give yourself time for a gradual transition – use the green tea or weak black tea option if you need to.

Cooked fatty foods seem to cause people to want very acid stimulating drinks to cut through and break down the greasy mess, and to keep them awake – hence the "supersize me" marriage between McDonalds, Coke and coffee. So in my humble opinion, drinks like Coca Cola, Pepsi and other canned and bottled sweet and fizzy drinks are quite simply appalling from a natural health perspective (and environmentally) and should be assigned to the past as soon as possible. Try the well-known experiment of putting a tooth or coin in a glass of Coke overnight! On the useful side, I've been told that diet coke makes a fantastic cleaner – but would you want to drink what's on the cleaning shelves at the supermarket? I have nothing more to say on these drinks, except that even those that masquerade as being healthy (i.e. 'diet this' or 'sugar free that') are normally not. The companies behind them could simply choose to create only the most health creating drinks possible, and put all their research and marketing might behind that - I suspect they'd get a vast and persistent wave of positive free publicity if they did ... may be one day!

Alcohol is for you to deal with as you see fit. It has a huge social role in western society. However, the plain fact is that it's one of the biggest killers and creators of illness and addiction, personal and family problems and unhappiness in our culture. More and more people are living with little or no alcohol, and having a great time without it. Your relationship with alcohol, if you have one, will probably evolve as you eat more raw. Red wine in smaller quantities is probably most acceptable from the raw perspective, ideally organic if bought, and even better would be home-made or locally made fruit wines from berries or other fruit such as plums. Local real ale or cider is the best option if you really love your pint, or want to carry on with it in social situations. From an environmental standpoint, depending on food miles, any alcohol made from fruit is generally better than one made from grain (because it means trees being planted and maintained, and soil undisturbed, rather high-input grain farming and soil compaction and erosion). And again, whatever it is go for organic of course, if you can.

LET'S BE HONEST, ARE THERE ANY DANGERS?

Yes, there are a few. However, to answer this properly, it's important to consider this question from a 'level playing field', that asks the same question of a conventional diet, and other diet choices like the Atkins approach. So let's not forget the very real dangers of a normal western diet. Look at the statistics and trends for health and the realities around you (e.g. for any over 50's and over 60's you know) that reflect the very predictable effects and significant dangers of a 'normal' diet first. Are there any dangers with that? Yes, there are many.

As with any diet or lifestyle, there are a few 'dangers', if that's the right word, with the completely raw lifestyle – but I don't believe there are any dangers with a 50% raw lifestyle, compared with a conventional diet. With an all / mainly raw diet some risks are physical, and some are emotional/psychological - but to me they are far fewer and less dangerous than sticking with the standard western diet. Risks can come from a) taking too rapid or too harsh an approach to cleansing, or b) an imbalanced, naively simplistic or extreme approach to the diet, which can lead to nutritional imbalances or deficiencies, or social isolation. But, from my experience, if a balanced approach is taken, with a good approach to cleansing, there are definite, significant benefits to the high raw / 100% raw path. And the risks are between 'far less' and 'non-existent' for a 50-80% raw diet - although many of the benefits may also be less, or slower to emerge.

For some people the risks of eating mainly / all raw can include social isolation - although raw gatherings, groups, networks, websites, blogs and magazines are often very vibrant, and can often even lead to a richer social life – as they did for many of my years of being raw. Raw food fundamentalism can be a danger for some. An unbalanced diet is the main danger, which can arise from eating too much hybridized food (fruit in particular), not getting enough greens and minerals in your diet, and particularly from B12 deficiency.

In more detail, some of the dangers include:

- **B12 Deficiency:** this is very important to be aware of and is mainly relevant to vegans, though not exclusively. My views on B12 evolved through my own experience and through observing other vegan raw food eaters over time. Vegans need to be aware of B12 deficiency, whether raw or not, so highly quality B12 supplements are recommended by most nutritionists, the Vegan Society, and so on. Whatever your diet, a vital issue with B12 is assimilation i.e. the B12 (and other nutrients) your body is able to take in through the digestive system, rather than the amount of B12 you consume. As well as B12 intake, this appears to depend on a) the alkalinity of your diet, as an over acid system inhibits B12 up-take, and b) how blocked and unhealthy your digestive system is, which is assisted by fasting, juice fasting, herbal cleanses or colonics. We need B12 for proper brain function, and it is essential for healthy pregnancy, so it is much better to take a B12 supplement or use some yeast extract in a salad or seed pate to avoid the risk of deficiency, especially in pregnant or nursing mothers and young children. B12 deficiency is not fun - with it you tend to feel 'all over the place', lost, disempowered and unable to focus or concentrate. So be aware of the potential for B12 deficiency and take specific action to avoid it. There is plenty of information about the B12 issue within the raw food and vegan networks, so you can always look into it more to help you make your own choice. Dr Gabriel Cousens is a particularly valuable source of information - see www.treeoflife.com. You don't need to be afraid of it – but you do need to be aware and make sure you take action and eat to avoid it. If you are going to have dairy, raw sheep's or goats cheese, yoghurt or milk are preferable.

- **Teeth:** Please ignore anyone who suggest you don't need to brush your teeth if you go all raw! We are all starting with non-ideal teeth, and usually from a lifetime of eating foods that are not good for the teeth. This means many people's teeth or gums are already not in great shape. Look after your teeth, and carry on brushing them, at least daily. Be careful about:

   a) Eating unripe fruit: particularly lots of unripe supermarket oranges (fresh and ripe from the tree is a different story!). With fruit, if it isn't ripe it's not good for the teeth, because it is more acid than nature intended it to be and the acid will attack the teeth and gums.

   b) Over-eating nuts: Frederic Paténaude, author of *Raw Secrets,* is convinced that there are dangers for the teeth from eating too many nuts, as this can create an acid environment in the mouth that eats away at the teeth and robs the body of minerals which would otherwise maintain your teeth and maintain the body's essential pH balance (I believe this theory is yet to be proven, but seems entirely logical). Fred recommends 100 grams max per day, soaked.

   c) Over-eating dried fruits: these are concentrated sugars, and as with any other concentrated sugar, excessive dried fruit can lead to teeth problems.

As with most things, balance is the key. And remember, a) the starches and sugars of a so called 'normal' diet are at least as much of a danger as the raw alternatives; b) eating plenty of fresh, organic greens (especially kale and wild foods) is good for your teeth and gum health.

- **Psychological Stuff:** An eat more raw lifestyle, if followed in a balanced way, will normally make you feel more alive, more healthy and more energized - but it is not a panacea that will automatically sort out the psychological and emotional problems (such as depression, eating disorders, ADHD, schizophrenia, etc) which are as widespread in our society as the physical health problems (such as obesity, cancer, heart disease, diabetes, etc). Over-eating and bad food combinations can be common when emotional issues arise, or when toxins come into the system leading to cravings to eat things that will stop the detox process. Limiting your fats and protein intake (i.e. nuts and seeds) is important, as over-acidity effects the emotions and raises stress levels. Eating an alkaline diet tends to calm and relax the body, mind and emotions. You may need to control a desire to over-eat, which is a desire to satisfy the appetite, and often to meet entirely unmet emotional needs, which have nothing to do with real hunger.[82] As previously stated *Raw Emotions* by Angela Stokes is very helpful in this area. For some, the more raw you go the more isolated from normal society you may feel, which can have its emotional and psychological challenges – networks, gatherings, magazines and so on all help with answers to the FAQ's and understanding the FEE's (Frequently Experienced Effects). As well as detoxing physically there is normally emotional detoxing that also goes on. So much depends on your character and personality, your awareness of these issues, your self awareness and your personal strength, as well as the support around you (or lack of it). Anyone needing psychiatric care or mental health support will probably get some benefits if they eat more raw and all organic (especially greens as they are the best source of minerals), particularly as research by the Behavioural Health Partnership and others suggests that many behavioural problems are directly linked to a lack of the essential vitamins and minerals which are needed for proper brain function. Anyone who is under Social or Mental Health Worker supervision will need to gain advice from a fully qualified nutritionist who has some awareness of the benefits of eating more raw (see contacts section in Appendices) – as they may face real challenges from the system if they are seen as fanatical or extreme. Going raw is not going to 'sort out' those psychological or emotional problems, although it may significantly help behavioural difficulties in children and adults (e.g. ADD and Hyperactivity, which are worsened by refined sugars, food additives, highly processed foods and chemicalised drinks). There are many influences and effects on our psychology and emotions of course, and many psychological and emotional problems go right back to childhood. Eating more raw foods can lift off some of the layers that 'dumb down' some of our patterns, and at the same time it can help us to see and experience things more clearly, so that we understand ourselves better and give ourselves more choices about how to respond to or change those patterns. Balance is the key, not extremism.

It is for you to decide whether the above issues are real 'dangers' or perhaps simply issues to be aware of and then to take sensible steps to avoid. Like a pot hole in the road when you're

---

[82] Marshall Rosenberg's NVC work can really help understand how to more effectively understand our feelings and meet our needs – see www.nonviolentcommunication.com or www.liferesources.co.uk

cycling, it can be dangerous if you are cycling in the dark, but if you have the light of awareness shining ahead of you it is a hole that is easy to avoid, *if you are looking where you are going.*

To me the clear reality is that the bigger dangers lie in cancers, heart disease, diabetes, obesity and other degenerative diseases, or rather in the causes of these degenerative diseases – in particular the standard western lifestyle and diet, which you should do your utmost to avoid or transform. Other significant dangers are apathy, ignorance and fear of change.

With a balanced *health creating diet*, shifting to anything from 50-100% raw, with some raw weeks each year, and /or several 3 day fasts each year, will certainly be a very positive change - if you cut out processed and fried foods, or drop or cut right back on "wheat, meat 'n' dairy", and other habits that are destructive for your health. Cutting right back on the bad stuff is making the pot holes smaller – it is not avoiding or getting rid of them.

SO WHAT ACTUALLY IS YOUR POSITION ON RAW FOODS?

My position? Well, I don't have a rigid position. I've felt good eating at least 50% fruit, and best eating daily salads picked fresh from the garden with a good variety of greens. I feel less good with a high intake of fat foods (avocados, oils, etc.) or high protein foods (nuts and seeds), particularly in a warm climate. A lot salty foods (like salted olives) do not make me feel good.

I have felt at my best eating simply - one or two types of fruit at a time during the day, with a salad in the late afternoon (in Spain) or evening (in England). I've also felt great eating only fruit for several days at a time, and have often felt excellent eating less for periods of time, particularly in a warm climate when I often only had water until around midday - but I would not recommend this at all if you are very active, new to raw food or a pregnant / nursing mother.

Eating more than we need is one of the main things that has greatly slowed or even blocked progress towards vibrant health for many on the 'eat more raw' path, myself included at times. But starvation diets are also a nutritional nightmare – to loose weight healthily you need excellent nutrition – which is well explained by Angela Stokes' e-books (www.rawreform.com).

If you want to follow a particular school of thought on your eat more raw path, many advocates of particular approaches are highly respected in the movement. You don't have to stick to one approach – but allowing any one approach enough time to be experienced properly is important, so try to avoid chopping and changing over short periods of time. Allow yourself time to transition, and over time trying different approaches may be important.

When you eat more raw and try different approaches it's good to really *feel the effects of your foods as you eat and digest them* - and feel the changes in your body as it cleanses. Listen to your body, listen to your emotions, listen to your mind and listen to your spirit – think about which of these are the most helpful guide at different times.

Don't pretend you are going all raw or mainly raw if you are not – decide on how raw you really want to be and do it. And then whether you are going completely raw or not, make sure you are not over-eating, and make sure you have a well-balanced diet. At least 50% raw fruits and vegetables, eating steamed or lightly boiled starchy vegetables as your cooked foods, with little or no grains, meat or dairy, and eating sensible and not excessive quantities will give you good, and possibly fantastic results.

One perspective that is shared amongst a group of natural health advocates was confirmed at a 'Raw Summit' in early 2006, where a set of core guidelines were adopted by 22 'raw leaders' with a combined total of 411 years experience of this diet. This group included Dr Brian and Anna Maria Clement, Dr Gabriel Cousens, Viktoras Kulvinskas, Jill Swyers, Paul Nison, Fred Bischi, Diana Store and others. The following statement is a summary of their guidelines:

The Optimum Diet for Health/Longevity:
Vegan (no animal products of any kind, cooked or raw)
Organic Whole Foods - High in nutrition such as vitamins, antioxidants and phytonutrients
Highly mineralized: contains a significant quantity of chlorophyll-rich green foods
Contains adequate complete protein from plant sources
Contains a large proportion of high-water content foods
Provides excellent hydration
Includes raw vegetable juices
Contains all essential fatty acids, including Omega 3 fatty acids from naturally occurring plant sources
Is at least 80% raw (the remaining to be Vegan, whole food, and organic)
Has moderate, yet adequate caloric intake
Contains only low to moderate sugar and exclusively from whole food sources (fruitarianism is strongly discouraged)
Is nutritionally optimal for both detoxification and rebuilding

We also agree that:
- Supplementation with Vitamin B-12 is advised.
- The addition of enzyme active superfoods and whole food supplements is also advised.
- This way of eating can be further optimized by tailoring it to individual needs (within the principles stated).
- Benefits derived by following these principles are proportional to how well they are followed.
- We will remain open-minded, and this information will be updated and expanded upon, if necessary, as new research becomes available.
- Diet is a critical piece of a healthy lifestyle, yet not the entire picture. A full spectrum, health supportive lifestyle is encouraged. This includes physical exercise, exposure to sunshine, as well as psychological health. Avoiding environmental toxins and toxic products is essential. Paramount is pure water (for consumption and bathing), the use of natural fiber clothing, and non-toxic personal care products. Also consider healthy options in home furnishings/building materials and related items.

All the attending leaders agreed that the main objective of eating in the above mentioned fashion is to promote health, and equally to prevent and minimize disease.[83]

---

[83] Source: www.rawsuperfoods.com

My own position focuses more on *why* and *how*, and less on the specifics of 'what'. I see numerous benefits arising from the eat more raw life, and suggest – as the raw leaders say – you find the individualised diet and balance that is the optimum for you. From my experience of living within the raw world and outside it, in the so called 'normal' world, most people aren't going to go for the all raw option, or the vegan option, even if evidence suggests it is the optimum diet for health and longevity. From where they are, such changes are one or several steps too far from what's normal to them, and how they live their life. Even so, to be aware of it, and to *see it as a possibility* some time may be very useful to you, even if you don't realise it now. Whatever level of transformation in diet, lifestyle and health you are seeking it will help you if you create your own *culture of change* – a culture which supports that transformation, rather than hinders it.

So I'm saying, be aware that it's an option. Most raw fooders are (of course) ordinary people who have made a major shift, often in just one part of their lifestyle. If the focus is on being practical and realistic rather than idealistic, then make what change you can, and aim for roughly 50% raw - or more raw than 50% if it feels right. That is realistic for most people. And as far as the benefits are concerned, some of the key ones can be easily summarised as follows, although they vary in strength according to the approach you follow:

12 REASONS TO EAT MORE RAW

1. Optimum health, energy and 'feel good' benefits
2. Powerful natural healing potential
3. Child and family health benefits
4. Ethics: ecological and compassionate benefits
5. Mental clarity and spirituality / consciousness benefits
6. Looking more beautiful, vital and with a healthy image
7. Seeing or enabling knock-on benefits in family, friends, relatives or work colleagues
8. Following intuition and simplification, creating more self-awareness
9. Cultural evolution – being part of a culture of change and a culture of health creation
10. Supporting positive businesses and creative economics
11. Personal liberation benefits and greater confidence in your health
12. Getting all the benefits together

And overall, a primary reason is that a healthy diet can be an extremely helpful contribution to living a positive life.

MAKING THE TRANSITION EASIER AND MORE SOCIAL

Make sure you plan in some significant milestones as targets, and for celebration:

1. Getting off processed foods
2. Reaching 50% raw
3. Maintaining 50% raw for a month

If you organize an *Eat More Raw Intro Workshop* (or something similar) you can then create a local support group who can get together to encourage, support and celebrate each other in making then changes, bringing a positive social dimension into the journey of transition.

PART 6: DESIGNING REAL HEALTH

THE TWELVE PETALLED FLOWER OF HEALTH

Whilst there is a lot more to food than meets the eye, there is also a lot more to health than diet or nutrition. So it's very important to consider the dimensions beyond diet, food and assimilation that contribute to a natural process of creating more complete, whole health for yourself and others. Overall 'real health' will arise naturally for individuals, families, communities or for a whole culture from bringing together the pieces of the whole health zigsaw puzzle, which work together beneficially to create real health. This is permaculture design of real health:

1. Health creating nutrition
2. Digestive health: healthy assimilation, elimination and detoxification
3. Exercise: Yoga, Five Tibetans, Tai chi, Aikido; walking, cycling, gym work or dance
4. Mental & spiritual health: meditation, spiritual practice/mental exercise & improvement
5. Positive communication e.g. using practices such as nonviolent communication (NVC)
6. Intimacy and physical contact e.g. loving intimate relationships, massage, etc
7. Friendship and community
8. Creativity and self-expression, plus laughter and enjoyment
9. Self-confidence: in physical and health terms, and in spiritual or psychological terms
10. Right livelihood: work that contributes to creation of health or sustainability
11. Sustainable living and healthy homes
12. Positive attitudes & a personal development path, towards whole health and fulfillment

To achieve 'Whole health' or 'Real Health', ideally all the above can work together – however, for many, realistically *3-6 of the above together will make a real health difference. This is also a realistic and achievable goal for most people – think about it for yourself.*

Physical exercise, relief of tension and body movement is required for excellent health. In particular it keeps the lymphatic system active and helps our breathing - as 60% of our energy is said to come from the air we breathe (via the burning of oxygen in our cells) this is very important. This is one reason why physically active people on a poor diet can maintain excellent fitness ... until they become less active, when they 'crash'. Then the effects of a bad diet often hits them hard, and suddenly they become ill.

As well as Yoga, The Five Tibetans, Tai Chi or Aikido (particularly the Ki school), dancing is excellent - and for the more physical and 'sporty' types the Royal Canadian Air Force 5BX programme was designed to get pilots to peak fitness with just 11 minutes of very carefully designed exercise per day.[84] Mike Nash's *Aggressive Health* is ideal for the fitness junkie who likes a lot of detail, combining a health creating diet with a powerful exercise regime.

---

[84] A small, neat book - *The Royal Canadian Air Force 5BX Programme*, Penguin (1986).

Deliberate exercise is an area in my life where I have not been consistent. I remain a generally active person, and in the past (up to my late 20's) playing a lot of sport, plus plenty of cycling and walking kept me generally fit. I have practiced Tai Chi and the Five Tibetans for extended periods with very significant effects, and now do yoga on a regular basis. I briefly dabbled with the 5BX programme, enough to know that it can generate high levels of fitness in a very short space of time.[85]

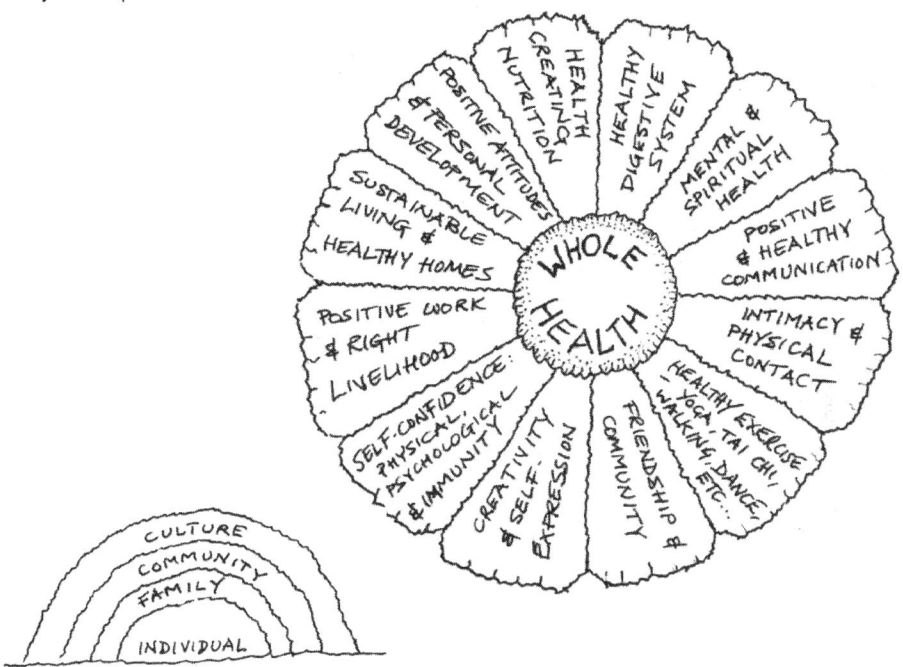

In a world which we are told is 'dangerous', where we are told to constantly fear attack and physical violence, learning some form of self-defense (physical and psychological) can help bring greater freedom in our lives, creating a feeling of greater self-confidence. Survival skills can also be very beneficial, building confidence that you can survive living simply in the great outdoors. Living very simply made a big difference to me, and for about for 5 years I lived close to nature, 'off-grid' without mains water and electricity – in a large ex-army tent, as part of a low impact healthy living project, with a beautiful river to bath in, and many other benefits from not having the things that most people consider essential, until they experience that they are not!

For me, going raw has strengthened my psychological confidence because I feel a strong immunity to normal humdrum illnesses. But, on the physical defense front I still need work. Aikido

---

[85] See the small and fascinating book *The Five Tibetans*, Christopher Kilham, Healing Arts Press (1994) – also *Just Eat An Apple*, Jan – Feb 2001 edition (issue 15) for an excellent summary by Fred Paténaude.

– 'The Way of Peace'- is a powerful form of self-defense - it does not teach attack. The Ki Aikido school emphasises nature, peace and harmony, as well as giving and mutual benefit –the dramatic and centering effect it has had on a good friend of mine has been obvious. To tackle and transform the challenges of the world and daily life, we need power but not aggression. Aikido and other spiritually-based martial arts are powerful parts of the personal web-of-health, bringing more confidence and direct positive action, as well as more health and joy into our lives.

In designing whole health, it can be a challenge to juggle the various balls in one's life and keep them going all together. It's a challenge to try to spin the complete web. Personally, I am not there and don't pretend to be. I have explored many of these elements in isolation and in combination with several others. As well as being all raw for lengthy periods, from time to time I have even managed seven or eight at the same time. These explorations have all had positive effects on my life, so I am hoping to share knowledge and enthusiasm, without giving myself a hard time for 'not being perfect', or not bringing all these elements together at the same time in my life consistently. I have made choices about my priorities, according to the time and the place I'm at in my life.

With significant life changes, it's often not a linear progression from one step to the next. What I see is a beautiful spider's web of health and sustainability, with each segment connected by any number of finely spun strands. You can enter into the web from any number of the 12 anchoring strands that connect it to the world it is a part of. Imagine such a web for yourself, where you might choose to enter, and what strands to your web you might have ... Imagine.

For example, you might find that gradually rising environmental or climate change concern leads you to an understanding of the interconnectedness of Earth Care – People Care – Fair Share issues ... which then may lead you to change your shopping, food buying and eating habits, for ethical and intellectual reasons. Then you may realize that health and ecological issues are intimately linked... leading you on to vegetarianism, veganism or raw food; doubling the amount of 'raw' in your life, and halving or cutting out the 'meat, wheat 'n' dairy' in your life.

With these changes you may discover it doesn't feel like you thought it would. In fact you find that it feels easy, positive and liberating. This then opens new doors for you... which you push wide open and stride through with greater confidence. It leads you to more understanding and empathy for yourself and others - which again feels good. So with a confident spring in your step and a smile on your face you start off down the personal development path. This in turn leads to yet more self-confidence, greater exploration and more life-changes, letting go of old blockages about what 'spiritual' means. So you freely choose to start to meditate... and a whole new world is opened up to you that you never realized existed before.

Just imagine a little longer how things can change, how one thing can lead to another... and how good that might feel.

All these life changes add up, and they can happen one by one, or in a cluster, creating positive ripple effects in the 'outside' world. You can start by passing through any one of these 'doorways'. Any one of them can lead you to other areas of discovery and growth. Like a stone thrown in a pond, the ripple effects can spread through your life and change your thinking and behaviour in other areas.

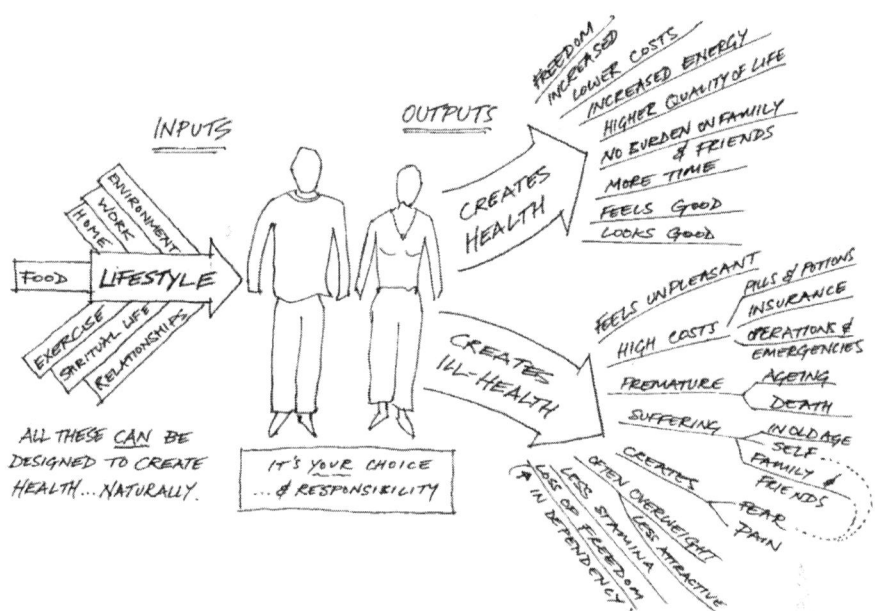

For me meditation was the doorway into all the other areas of concern – where some doors were ajar, suddenly they started flying open. This led to a raised level of general awareness, with my underlying interest in nature growing into fully blown environmental concern, with an eco-spiritual seed sown which has grown strongly ever since. My opening eyes led me to do a 2 week permaculture design certificate course back in '94 where, by chance, I met a knowledgeable and experienced raw fooder (when few of these were about!). Being an ecologically minded vegan already, that got me into the raw food thing. In turn all these things led me to want to live in a health conscious ecological community, with like-minded others, sharing similar concerns and visions. That created Ecoforest, which helped hundreds of people to experience a different kind of life. What I came to see through Ecoforest was that the changes in my life then directly enabled and created significant positive changes in other people's lives … which then directly enabled and created significant positive changes in yet more people's lives … and so it goes on … the ripple effects flow on and on, even now.

The spider's web we each weave is the heart of our own personal 'web of life'. Each web has interconnected segments for your diet, shopping patterns, your work, exercise, meditation, food growing and so on. And your web is connected to a wide chain of effects in the outer world. It's also connected to a chain of effects in the inner world of mind, body, emotions and spirit. The web of internal effects is connected to the web of external effects. All these aspects of your life you can design to be mutually beneficial as part of a personal plan to redesign or fine tune your life.

So if you want to change the world, and to experience whole health, you have to start by changing and respinning your own web of life.

MEDITATION

Meditating is a perfect complement to a better diet and a more ecological lifestyle. Meditation can be part of your daily diet that will help bring a more complete level of physical, mental, emotional and spiritual health. Learn to meditate from a good teacher, with regular support, encouragement and advice for at least the first three months after learning. Otherwise you may be left with unanswered questions and queries as the meditation starts to take effect, and as your perception and experience of life changes. With meditation, the learning of the technique is normally fairly simple. It's the consistent practice in the first month or two that is the key to success, and the main challenge. Like eating more raw, establishing a new timetable in your daily life is sometimes easy, and sometimes hard.

Starting to meditate as part of a completely new pattern in life can work well (like a change in diet). From my own experience I can recommend TM (Transcendental Meditation) as a technique, although it may not be right for everyone. From experience I know it can be incredibly powerful and effective – and I mean 'incredible' in the literal sense, which is that it is not credible to the logical mind; the logical mind cannot accurately understand or imagine the effects. TM took me to a state of being in my everyday life that was very positive, stress-free and creative, opening me up to see that I was not who I thought I was. So it really helped me to evolve in a very positive way. Generally, it is not cheap to learn TM - but in my experience if you keep it up it will repay you many times over, in many different ways. Be aware that some teachers have broken free of the main TM movement (i.e. The Meditation Trust, UK), particularly to make the technique available to more people at affordable prices.

Whether it's politics, religion, a sport, TM or the natural health movement, there are always people that like to identify themselves with one particular idea, movement, way of life or practice. This is more a reflection of people than anything to worry about with TM or eating more raw food. We all have huge potential, and the frightening challenge is to face up to being your own guru, learning from a range of sources. Meditation can be a very positive and healthy part of your life, and it's worth noting that the TM movement has been responsible for a vast amount of respected scientific research into the effects of meditation.

TM only takes about 40 to 50 minutes a day (about 20 minutes each in the morning and evening). I slept less, but much better and this meant I did things much more effectively - so I gained far, far more than those 40 to 50 minutes spent meditating. The now world-famous Dr Deepak Chopra emerged through the TM movement and his early works are good sources of information about the beneficial effects of TM and the practice.

My own experiences with meditation included internal travels to places of freedom, openness and a kind of expansive joy that I had no idea existed beforehand. And there is no question that this had profound and positive effects on the way I interacted with people and the world. So I know that the idea of the 'discipline' of meditation, twice a day, for a period of many years is just an idea – it is not how it was for me. I meditated every day, twice a day for eight years, with no problem doing so even when I was traveling. Even on a coach or a train I could easily sit quietly and go to deep, expansive and relaxing spaces.

Vipassana is another powerful meditation technique that many of my friends have explored with significant and extremely positive results. Vipassana seems to work very well as a way of moving through some big internal challenges, gaining profound insights and helping to change your life for the better. Following it up after the initial retreat requires a commitment of time (one to two hours a day) – everyone I know who has kept this up says it has paid them huge dividends although many don't succeed with maintaining the core practice because it is a big commitment of time. The philosophy of Vipassana is admirable, as those doing a retreat need not pay, but are encouraged to make a donation according to the value they feel they have received or work as helpers on future retreats.

Through friends, I also know that breathing and body conscious Buddhist and yoga meditations are also very clarifying and stabilising, and are used by many to great effect. Martial arts related meditations and dynamic meditations such as Tai Chi can also be very powerful, as can those used in Kundalini Yoga. Allowing the mind to follow the breath or the sensations of the body, takes it out of its mental sphere – which is the primary objective of meditation.

My experience of TM is that it seems to 'hypnotise' the left brain, allowing the right brain to be more fully and directly experienced, providing wholly different experiences and insights to those that dominate our day-to-day life. But understanding how it works is not the important thing... experiencing it, doing it is the important thing. In reality, once you've got the initial pattern going, and start to reach some deeper states, consistent meditation is usually relatively easy, very rewarding and something to look forward to every day.

A common theme in meditation teaching is to encourage students not to mix techniques. This is good advice. Various meditation techniques have been developed because they are effective. They work in different ways to shift us to different states of experience. Thousands of years of observation and practice sit wisely behind most of these techniques. I believe it is worth breaking through our limiting and often somewhat brattish, western ideas of what freedom is. These often emerge in our minds as 'I can do whatever I want, when I want, and I don't have to do it that way if I don't want to!'

My experience is that this attitude is a huge trap. In reality there is more freedom in finding we have choice even within structured and consistent practices – 'I can choose to follow strict guidelines and be utterly free in that choice'. Without feeling we are giving up our freedom, power or control of our lives, we can find that a little 'order' in our lives, and respect for ancient principles, can take us to sources and places of freedom we cannot even imagine.

The same goes for when you eat more raw. I have heard so many times people say that "it must take so much discipline"... It's quite the reverse for me. In fact, once the first life changes are made, and new patterns established, it can be a massive liberation. Most meditation schools have their own ideas about diet, mainly promoting vegetarianism, as well as simple eating and fasting for advanced practices. I see natural and complementary benefits in combining more raw foods with meditation. So I feel that any positive change in your lifestyle or diet is likely to deepen your experience of meditation... and vice versa; meditation is only likely to enhance any other positive lifestyle or diet changes you make.

POSITIVE MENTAL AND SPIRITUAL NUTRITION

A brief word on positive mental and spiritual nutrition feels important. I have certainly found it really good for my mental and spiritual health to remind myself to *"Programme yourself with positivity, health and sustainability"*.

The media and 'health system' tend toward a disempowering view that tells us it's 'natural' for us to become seriously ill. Sometimes I feel angry about this, at other times sad - because I believe it is not true, and because many, many human beings experience a huge amount of unnecessary suffering because of this cultural belief in the normality of illness. It also has a massive social, emotional and economic costs – and is a monumental waste of human potential. No one in particular is to blame for this cultural belief, because so many parts of our socio-economic and cultural jigsaw puzzle support and buy into the belief. It's a well-established pattern, and a well-established belief; even an understandable belief... but that does not make it true, wise or justifiable.

Yes, it is now 'normal' for people to get seriously ill, but it is certainly not natural – and it's not a positive or helpful attitude to be resigned to this idea. From experience I also believe it is not necessary for most people to get seriously ill either, given enough information, time, support and confidence in our lives. A more holistic, truly scientific and ecological understanding of health, and a clearer feel for what health and nature actually is can be very positive and helpful. We all have the potential to replace the old belief with a better informed, more positive and more helpful belief – including many people who are seriously ill, as the second half of Part Eight of this book shows. So to be really effective in changing your own life for the better you need to close off the taps that keep that negative flow pouring in, and open up the channels that allow a more positive flow of information and inspiration to flood into your life. Instead of watching television and buying newspapers which sell the same old drag-me-down messages, change what you feed your mind and spirit on.

To get your positive flow going: subscribe to *Permaculture Magazine, Funky Raw Magazine, Vibrance* eZine, *Get Fresh, Positive News* or other positive publications.[86] Buy books that bring you new, positive and helpful information. This will allow you to grow and develop organically. Become part of an active, positive network or some kind of group of friends with a common positive and/or creative interest. Explore new activities, be courageous and take the adventurous route that your heart and intuition tell you to. Take some chances, play and explore - mix with active, positive networks of people of like mind.

It is also useful to recognise that our language and culture is full of restricting or negative subconscious programming. Changing the patterns of words you use, will change the way you think, and changing the way you think will change the way you act. A simple example of this is that we always have a choice to say something other than 'yes' or 'no'. So when someone presents me with a narrow 'either/or' choice, I find it much more creative and realistic to think of a third option... because nature always offers us much more than just an 'either/or' choice.

---

[86] *Living Nutrition Magazine* was published from 1996 to 2008, and since then it has been reborn as *Vibrance* eZine, published electronically by Living Nutrition LLC – see http://www.livingnutrition.com/

PROGRAMME YOURSELF WITH POSITIVITY, HEALTH AND SUSTAINABILITY

Protesting against the things we don't believe in has a positive role.

However, being mainly 'against' things is a trap that keeps all those negative things dominant in your mind. For me it gave no space to create the positive alternatives.

If we want new, more positive things to happen, we have to shift the majority of our attention and action to creating those positive alternatives.

If we really follow the *'Be the change you want to see in the world'* (Gandhi) doctrine it will naturally lead us to create more positive, naturally healthy and sustainable lives. It's important to get the balance right, with up to a third of your energy going into protest if you wish, but *ensure that at least two thirds of your action, thoughts and energy (including your work) goes into creating the positive life and the positive world that you want and feel is needed for yourselves and future generations.*

This should be a fundamental guide in the personal politics of positive action. No one else is going to do it for you (or us); we have to actually create it ourselves, and not just protest about what we don't want. So be the change you want to *be* in the world. *Create the alternatives.*

Understanding and acting on this is absolutely fundamental - because if we do not do it, then the creative power of what comes next in the world and in our lives stays with those we are protesting against, or simply complaining about if we haven't been active enough to protest. This is the most important and most significant shift in power that needs to be put in place, the power of creating the future from the present. This is about establishing a positive, healthy, sustainable culture of change.

'Take Responsibility For Yourself' and recognise your own power in any and every situation. Use tools to explore where you're heading in your life and where you really want to be. Recognise that you have changed and you will change. Create the possibility of real health for yourself and then identify and take the practical first steps that will change your life positively. Keep identifying and taking the practical next steps. Plan and implement your own positive and effective personal transformation towards a more healthy, sustainable and fulfilling lifestyle. This means getting on and doing it. Book yourself on a permaculture course and raw food workshop – go on, you've got nothing to loose and everything to gain.

If you are in a relationship, doing this exploration with your partner or family can be tremendously creative, satisfying, supportive and enjoyable. However, also be open to entering into the adventure of life change on your own or with a wider group of friends, to discover new ways of doing things that provide mutual support and fun.

Just reading about these steps to change your life will have some small effect. And taking one or two steps as a result will create a ripple effect of change. Taking at least four or five steps will really start things moving positively though!

A 6 Month to 1 Year Outline Plan

- Stage 1: Alkalise and rehydrate i.e. eat plenty of fresh greens and alkalizing foods, remove and reduce acidifying foods, use alkalizing supplements (such as Marine Minerals supplements, green leaf powders via funkyraw.com, Detox Trading, E3Live, Nature's First Food, etc), drink more water and fresh juice. Get to 50% raw.
- Stage 2: Detoxify and cleanse the digestive and assimilation systems and the body as a whole e.g. Arise and Shine or Ejuva herbal cleanses; Sura Retreats cleansing retreats; short fasts; liver/gall bladder and kidney cleanses; parasite cleanse.
- Stage 3: significant juicing.
- Stage 4: rebuild and regenerate with greens and nutrient-dense foods; superfoods and supplements; and high quality fats.
- Stage 5: stabilize diet with top quality nutrition for body and brain.
- Stage 6: continue with a programme of short annual cleanses.

Routes and costs:
- The costly route: book yourself on retreats, workshops, seminars and supervised cleanses.
- The cheaper route: self-managed, read books to inform yourself first, use home-sprouting, grow much more of your own foods, drink more water and use wild greens juices (e.g. nettles), meet up and support/be supported by others on a similar path (e.g. via Funky Raw mag / events), etc.
- Mid-cost route: a mixture of the above options.

Vision and Practical First Steps:
- Develop a vision or accept the possibility of yourself as a vibrantly healthy person or with significantly improved health; see yourself living a highly sustainable lifestyle.
- First Practical Steps: define your holistic path to health, involving a continuing cycle of learning and taking action and learning and taking action e.g.:
    - Your Juice Month;
    - Your Greens Month;
- Your Action-Learning Group: get together with 2-5 other people on a similar path, comparing and contrasting your experiences, learning from and with each other, and having fun along the way – each time you meet share with each other a) what's going well, b) what's challenging, c) your vision for the next month (three months or year), and d) your practical next steps.

USE THESE TOOLS TO HELP YOU

Use the following tools to help you on your path:

- ☐ **Remove Limiting Factors:** what's limiting your progress or enjoyment, and how can it be removed or reduced?

- ☐ **Adding Creative Factors:** what new factors, activities or elements will support or accelerate your progress? What actions will unleash positive change in your life?

- ☐ **PMI: 'Plus Minus and Interesting'** – what's positive, what's negative and what's interesting about the journey, new experiences or lifestyle change?

- ☐ **Zones, Sectors and Slope:** what 'zones' of your life are you spending most time and energy on? From which sectors of the outside world do relevant information and other resources come to you? What makes you feel like you are sailing downhill? And what's an uphill struggle?

- ☐ **Attitude principles:** work with attitude principles to help your transition – e.g. a) working with the nature of yourself, and with the nature of your body's innate intelligence; b) turning a key problem or challenge into a solution, by understanding the deeper nature of the problem; c) make small changes to create big effects in your life; d) everything gardens, e) yield is unlimited, f) harvest only sunshine.

- ☐ **Questions to answer every week:** these are widely used in permaculture action-learning, setting aside an hour or so to ponder them and write them down:

    - What's Going Well? ....
      ....

    - What's Challenging? ....
      ....

    - What have I particularly liked? ....
      ....

    - What will I do differently? ....
      ....

    - What's my Vision or my possibility for the next month/week? ....
      ....

    - What are my Practical Next Steps toward my Vision for the next week?
      ....
      ....

PART 7: THE ROLE OF PERMACULTURE

So what is the role of permaculture in all this? What is its role in improving the quality of our nutrition and in transforming our lifestyle in order to create health?

The point of bringing permaculture into our work on natural health is reflected by the insight that underlies the *Real Health* philosophy - which is that real health in any part of a system can only be created if the whole system is healthy. So *individual health can only be created at its deepest level if the local-to-global system we are part of is healthy and naturally health creating.* Therefore *designing and creating naturally health creating human habitats* has to be fundamental to any wise approach to *environmental and human health creation*, which goes beyond just the 'me' mindset and attitude.

In addition to this there are two particular points about the role of permaculture in all this – one coming from the theory side, and the other from the totally practical side.

Firstly, in many ways there's a hidden hypothesis in this book – which is that:

If anyone truly applies the ethics, principles and practices of permaculture, or action-based approach to natural ecological thinking and design, to whole health, diet, natural nutrition and lifestyle then the most logical conclusion (and imperative) is the 'eat more raw' lifestyle.

Equally, if anyone truly 'gets' the deeper understanding of natural nutrition, and the supreme intelligence of nature and its pursuit of health, they should be growing food for themselves using permaculture systems, and be supporting ecological food supply chains.

Secondly, on the practical side, the most vital, nutritious foods are those eaten completely fresh. So growing and eating your own fresh food really does make a great deal of difference – even if it's just a little, but more so if it's a lot. So if you're looking to change and improve your diet and you're not already growing some of your own food then I encourage you to start growing some when changing your diet. And if you really understand the underlying reasons why eating more raw is beneficial, then you should also really understand the benefits of growing and eating more home-grown food, and act on that, even if it is on a small scale. And if you don't understand it yet, then contemplate it for a while longer, and contemplate through trying it.

In essence, permaculture is simply a way of embodying the principles and practices of nature – or the laws of nature - into a form of thinking and a practical system that we humans can apply to our lifestyles, the way we grow food, what we eat, and how we live. A practical example of this thinking is a 'fedge' - or 'food producing hedge' (i.e. fruits plus hedge-row salad plants such as hedge garlic) - is also a boundary, a sun-trap/wind break and a wildlife habitat, as well as a teacher and a thing of beauty. A forest garden is a multi-layered food producing system and a wonderful example of permaculture thinking and practice. For example, through careful design of a forest garden you can:

- protect and improve the soil and water resources;
- create a diverse supply of foods, timber and other outputs (fibre, medicines, etc);
- create an excellent habitat for wildlife;
- create a partially self-managing ecosystem - with plants, insects and other wildlife working together to meet each other's needs.

These are simple examples of permaculture thinking that are explained in more detail in the coming pages. The key point to get across is that permaculture is most easily learnt by applying its philosophy and techniques to our gardens, food growing systems and our homes. However, its principles, thinking and tools *are equally relevant and powerful if applied to our health.* So the following pages are intended to give you a feel for permaculture thinking, and are intended to expand the way you apply it in your life.

THE IDEA AND PRACTICE OF CREATING MANY BENEFITS

Permaculture empowers us to take greater control of our lives. It can be applied at the level of the individual, the household, the neighbourhood / community or the farm. It takes knowledge of self-seeding plants, perennial vegetables, fruiting trees and shrubs, herbs, companion planting, soil life, energy efficiency, composting, ponds, ground cover plants, climbing plants, water use, waste, renewables and appropriate technology, ecological building and much more, and gives you a method of enabling them to work together. Wherever permaculture is applied, a basic principle is to seek to create several benefits at the same time - not just one.

Whether you have a window sill or balcony, a medium-size garden, or a thousand acre farm, permaculture helps get more out, putting less in. It offers real opportunities to create healthy, sustainable lifestyles and living environments in urban, semi-urban and rural situations.

And permaculture thinking and design can help in any aspect of your lifestyle - physical, mental, emotional and spiritual nutrition, health and personal development. It involves developing the skills of working with nature, by generating a sense of interconnectedness, mutual-benefit and oneness. It sees everything that you are part of as a single extended system of trees, herbs, insects and wildlife - all working together for the health of the whole system, through living relationships. It is not a 'fluffy' perspective. Permaculture can be used in a very scientific or engineering-minded way too, to great effect. In fact, such an approach has massive potential. When you sense nature's diversity, dynamic stability, intelligence, abundance and creativity you can start to really work with that to create true health and sustainability.

So if you apply permaculture thinking in a concerted way to health, nutrition and your lifestyle then you'll probably end up significantly healthier.

LEARNING ABOUT PERMACULTURE: THE ETHICS AND DESIGN PRINCIPLES

From this point on, this chapter explains the foundations of permaculture whilst also demonstrating how those foundations can be applied to natural health and nutrition, at the same time as applying them to creating real health in ecological, social or economic terms. The starting point in permaculture is it's three ethics of *Earth Care*, *People Care* and *Fair Shares* – and the objective of designing solutions where all these three ethics meet.

There's a nice progression in the foundations of permaculture from three ethics to six attitude principles to twelve design principles. You don't need to remember them all, you just need to remember to use them regularly and that *they are here in this book whenever you need them.* The more you use them in your life, the more easily you remember them, and eventually you start to use them naturally and automatically without even thinking about it.

Three Ethics
1. *Earth Care:* looking after the planet's needs, and the local ecology.
2. *People Care:* looking after human needs – physical, social, economic and psychological.
3. *Fair Share:* of resources for people and planet, limits to consumption and sharing surplus.

Six Attitude Principles
1. *The Problem Is The Solution:* understand the deeper nature of the problem, to turn problems to solutions and liabilities to assets.
2. *Maximum Output for Minimum Effort / Small Changes for Bigger Effects:* small changes increase output, more than added input; the effect should be greater than effort;
3. *Work With Nature:* nature knows best; learn from and work *with* nature, not against it, to increase yields and benefits, outside and inside.
4. *Everything Gardens:* everything works to create the environment it needs; every element has some effect in the system, so work with the effects positively.
5. *The Yield Is Theoretically Unlimited:* increase the yield quantity/quality; notch up yield in subtle ways, and see/create gardens / lifestyles as multidimensional ecosystems.
6. *Harvest Only Sunshine (Closing The Loop):* use only renewable resources, and be positive in your thoughts and actions. Create 'closed loop' systems.

Twelve Technical Design Principles
1. *Relative location:* think about how each element or process is placed in relation to others, so that each element meets another's needs and uses other elements' outputs.
2. *Multi-use (the three-use rule):* make sure every element or process you design in is multi-functional, with at least three uses.
3. *Multi-supply:* meet needs from various sources - 'don't put all your eggs in one basket'.
4. *Energy efficient planning: zones, sectors and slope* – see following pages.
5. *Accelerated succession:* speed up nature's natural processes of growth, diversification and enrichment, nutrient recycling, fertility and diversity.
6. *Cycling of energy and resources:* seek to cycle energy, nutrients, water and resources within your system to raise productivity and diversity of yields.
7. *Biological resources:* use biological where ever possible to meet your needs and the needs of your 'pc system'.
8. *Diversity:* follow the pattern of nature, which is that diversity => multi-function + multi-supply + dynamic stability + productivity + resilience.
9. *Small scale intensive systems:* these systems are most productive - 'start at your backdoor and work out on a controlled front'.
10. *Edge effect:* the edge between ecosystems is usually most productive (e.g. the pond or woodland edge) – use this effect, create 'edge' in appropriate places to raise productivity.
11. *Appropriate technology:* use technology that is environmentally, financially and culturally appropriate, which is easily maintained, affordable and repairable. Simple is often best.
12. *Stacking in space and time:* use vertical space to create multi-level systems that give harvests throughout the year – epitomized by forest gardening, which is described in the next few pages.

Four 'permaculture soundbites' can also be really helpful to remember and apply:

a) "Unused outputs = pollution" i.e. you need to 'work' to remove any output that is not used by another element of the system.
b) "Unmet needs = work" i.e. you need to work to meet any needs of an element that are not met by the output of another element.
c) "No bare soil" i.e. any plant, even a 'weed', helps to protect the soil from sun and rain, and to build up the life and fertility of the soil, so no space should be left with bare soil. Maintaining bare soil involves work, and for good reason, nature does not leave soil bare.
d) 'There's no such thing as waste in nature' – every output is used by something else (this one should be starting to sink in by now!).

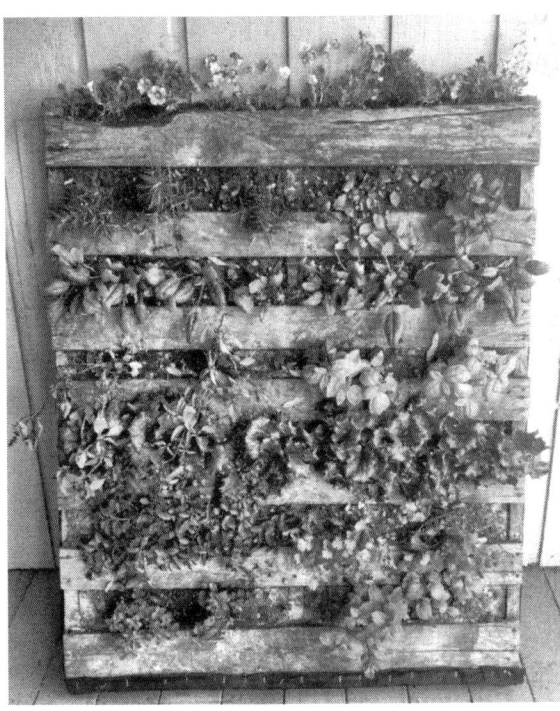

A pallet garden is an example of permaculture in practice, where a small space can be used for creating some meaningful productivity, with few resources – in an attractive and enjoyable way.

The basics are:

1. Prepare pallet so that the soil will stay in place
2. Plant-up the pallet on the horizontal
3. Let roots grow into soil/compost
4. Move pallet to vertical

There's plenty of information on the internet to show you how to make a pallet salad garden, and much more.

PERMACULTURE DESIGN TOOLS AND STRATEGIES

'Zones, Sectors and Slope' is another name for the technical principle of **efficient energy planning** and aims for more productive use of the energy that is stored in the site, and which flows through it. There are two types of zoning: **Site Zones** and **Bioregional Zones**.

Zones

Site Zones are used in permaculture as a flexible tool to increase efficiency in what we do, and the way we live. Site Zones look at where and how we expend our energy / work and concentrate this in central zones, working outwards to less active zones. The typical site-based zoning system considers the site, plot or area which is being worked with or designed, and works from Zone 0 to Zone 5. Zone 0 is inside the home, building or centre of activity, such as a school. Zones 1 and 2 are *the intensive gardening zones* immediately around the house or centre of activity, from where we move out through the other zones to Zone 5 at the edge.

- **Zone 0** is **indoors**, and normally is where we spend most time, where we are most active, where most attention is focused and most energy is used. Designing Zone 0 is vital, looking at inputs and outputs, activities and so on, to make Zone 0 healthy and productive.

- **Zone 1** is **immediately outside** and around the home (school, office, etc) and for a house is normally mainly for all-year salad and herb cultivation, with those plants that need most attention and energy input, plants which leaves will be picked from virtually every day, climbers, small shrubs, a pond (however small) and maybe some dwarf trees or trained trees on the wall, a fence or some other vertical element. Rainwater collection is also common in Zone 1.

- **Zone 2** is for other vegetables, soft fruit and fruit trees, and normally for a main composting system, where these elements need less than daily energy input and attention, making it the main forest gardening or food forest zone.

- **Zone 3** is the main crop area (e.g. potatoes, etc) visited less often, or the commercial zone, and area of extensive horticulture, agriculture or the agroforestry zone – or all of these.

- **Zone 4** is for **managed woodland** and forest.

- **Zone 5** is **wilderness** - unmanaged, undisturbed land, a place to observe, learn and enjoy, where nature and wildlife are left to do as they wish.

This is a flexible system, with the shape and size of zones adjusted to the landscape and situation – for example, you won't have much Zone 4 in a suburban garden or the backyard of a terraced house! Ponds are particularly valuable in Zones 1 and 2, as are climbers – whether they are grape vines, sugar snap peas, runner beans, passion fruit, Siberian kiwi or cultivated blackberries. In Zone 3 larger ponds, or even lakes and reservoirs, may be relevant.

Zoning helps structure your thinking during the design stage. It suggests that - unlike the traditional garden - you <u>don't</u> put the veg garden and compost heap at the far end of a long garden plot where you can only see what's going on if you're there, and which requires trudging down to on a wet and windy autumn or winter afternoon. Instead you put your salads, herbs, veg, soft fruit and compost system much closer, near the backdoor and visible from the house, where they will naturally get more and better attention – which automatically means it is more productive. And you can easily integrate flowers into the veg beds both for their own beauty, because many are delicious to eat and for their benefits with pollination and for attracting pest predator insects.

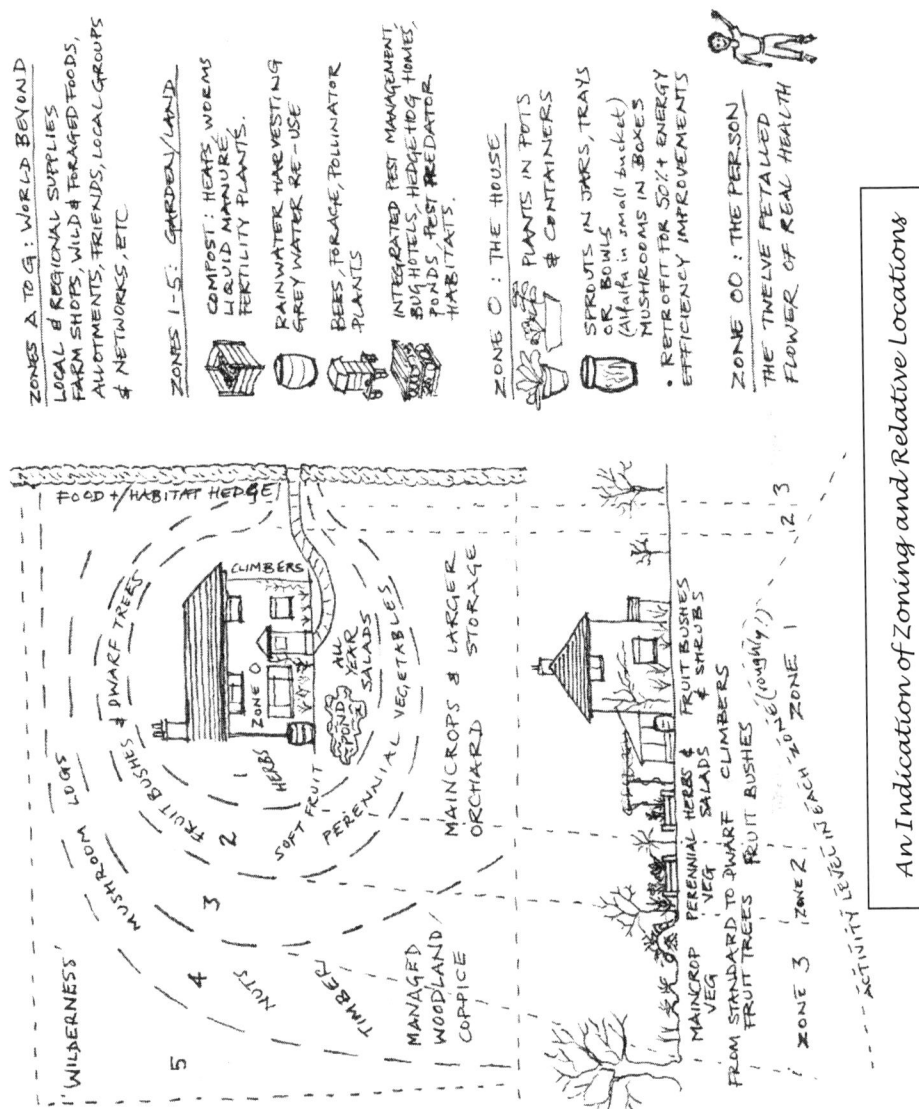

An Indication of Zoning and Relative Locations

Bioregional Zoning

Bioregional Zoning is a zoning system which considers our activities and impacts beyond the house and plot – in particular it provides a rough target for the degree of needs we meet from each zone. This is particularly useful for a wider sense of what sustainable living means in practice, in our relationships with the wider world. In this system Zones A to G cover:

A. The site i.e. house / building and grounds, farm, small-holding, etc (i.e. Zones 0-5).
B. The immediate environment, neighbourhood or local settlement.
C. The district/town (or municipality).
D. The bio-region.
E. The country as a whole.
F. The global region (e.g. Europe, north America, Australasia).
G. The Earth, the planet as a whole – so G is for Gaia, or the Globe as a whole.

The practicalities of sustainable lifestyle design with Zones A to G are:

Zone	Needs Met		Where & What
A	50%	If 0%	**The Site (Zones 0-5):** aim for *at least 50%* of needs to be met within this zone e.g. food needs, social needs, security, energy, etc.
B	25%	50%	**The Neighbourhood / Community:** at least 75% of needs from Zones A + B e.g. more food, energy and social needs, etc.
C	12%	25%	**The Municipality:** ideally approx 87% of needs from zones A-C e.g. work needs, most energy, food, education, most leisure, health etc.
D	6%	12%	**The Bioregion:** ideally approx 93% of needs from zones A-D e.g. construction needs, higher education and research, some leisure and energy, specialist health. And if 0% of needs can be met in Zone A, for example for someone who is very ill, 87% of needs are met by A-D.
E	3%	6%	**The Nation or State** in US/Canada /Australia, etc: at least 96% of needs from zones A-E.
F	2%	3%	**The Global region** (e.g. W Europe): >98% of needs from zones A-F.
G	1%	2%	**Gaia / the Globe**, the planet as a whole: >99% of needs from A-G.
			Which leaves up to 1% of needs being met from cosmic sources of supply!

In the permaculture courses I teach, this zoning system helps people gain a sense of context, for their life beyond the home, and gain a meaningful sense of what sustainability means in practice. It gives permaculture's Zones 0 to 5 a context and a connection with the locality, the bioregion and beyond, so that you can see the local-to-global picture as a whole.

This is a flexible model, to be used as a rough guide. However, after years of work on local to national sustainability projects, and grassroots permaculture, the figures it provides for the proportion of needs to be met from within each band of Zones are practical, easy to understand

and generally realistic. It works well as a practical guide for people wanting to look at how to transform their impacts by focusing on how they meet their needs – or more simply, how and where they spend their energy and money.

Basically, if the local to bioregional levels (Zones A to D) are sorted, most of the rest is. So, if 85-95%+ of your needs are met within the BioRegion you are living a pretty sustainable life. This should include social, education and leisure needs, food, energy and other essentials. For example, until relatively recently in building our homes and towns, virtually all our building needs were met at the local or bioregional level, and led to regionally distinct styles of building. It's one area that could shift relatively easily, both in the design and the performance of buildings if we evolve our thinking, learning from the excellent examples of ecological design and building that already exist.[87] Needs for information, higher education, business and social networks, research and so on are other areas that are very well met at the bioregional level.

In terms of Transition Town[88] thinking for example, our energy needs are currently met from remote regional or national power generation, through large power stations and the national grid. A transition to sustainable energy systems means creating a balanced mix of renewable energy generation in Zones A (home / on-site generation), B (neighbourhood / near-site generation), C (local / municipal generation) and D (regional generation) with the proportion of generation within these zones depending on the particular situation. (Plus much higher efficiency of course!)

Thinking in terms of these zones helps to change your consumer impacts in a significant and positive way. Thinking about diet runs from Zone G to Zone 00, the one zone not yet mentioned. **Zone 00** is the person, and in many ways *this is a book about design in Zone 00* – one of the first. Diet has huge implications for so many aspects of lifestyle, within your living space and with major implications across Zones A to G.

For example, humanity's use of just five crops – wheat, maize, rice, soya and potatoes – to supply more than 50% of its global food consumption is directly linked to the typical diets people eat. All these mono-crops, apart from some types of maize (which is deeeee-licious raw), need to be cooked (though you can sprout some rice and wheat). If you change what you eat and how you obtain it, you can change the inter-connected chain of effects in all these zones, from Zone 00 to Zone 5, and from Zone A to Zone G. Think about that and then intelligently design some positive changes to benefit yourself, others and nature/the earth as a whole.

An eat more raw diet is essentially a matter of designing the designer. And as all design comes from the designer (Zone 00) it seems particularly sensible to design for health and productivity in that part of the overall system. 'Real Health' is about the design of Zone 00 and its interconnections out through all the zones to Zone G.

---

[87] See www.sustainablehousing.org.uk or www.aecb.net if you are interested in green building and design. Also www.carbonlite.org.uk if you are interested in designing ultra low energy buildings.

[88] This model can be of value to the Transition Town movement, which is a good focus for communities responding practically to climate change & sustainability issues i.e. for considering the 'energy descent plan'. A need in the Transition movement is for adaptable, replicable models for creating and growing local social enterprises that are focused on a) energy efficiency and renewable supply (ESCo's), b) low carbon refurb and sustainable building, and c) local food production and distribution – but that's another book.

Sectors

Sectors are used to take advantage of energy flows into and through your site:
- Sunshine and light: the sunny or shady sectors of your site, the winter sunrise and sunset, and the summer sunrise and sunset;
- Winds and shelter: prevailing winds or strong cold winds – windy / sheltered sectors;
- Wet and dry: any water which flows or stands in your site – the wet / dry sectors;
- Fire, noise and other influences: fire risk sectors in warmer climates, neighbours, sources of pollution, etc.

Sectors help you place things in the landscape to make the most of the sun, shelter, water and so on, and help you to use that to best effect. Times of day and seasons of the year can be seen as sectors in time. During each day we go through various cycles. In terms of diet, for me this has meant I have a different balance of raw foods depending on what sector of the day or year I am in; with heavier foods such as nuts in winter and lighter fruit in summer... following nature's patterns.

Slopes

Slopes aim to be used to best advantage in permaculture – slopes that face the sun, cooler, shaded slopes, sheltered slopes and where frost pockets may lie. This is about using gravity and orientation. Slopes can be used to reduce work, for example by planting timber trees at the top of the slope, so that when they are harvested they only have to be moved down hill – or regeneration with self-seeding plants sited uphill, so that they spread their seeds easily and naturally downhill over time. On a smaller scale this also works by sowing self-seeding salad plants at the top (like rocket or hedge-garlic), with gravity, aided by the movement of water, moving the seeds down the slope over time. Slope is vital for using, holding and moving water for maximum benefit, including movements of water below the ground surface.

When you see and think in terms of zones, sectors and slopes you sense the microclimates on your site. This enables you to select and design in activities, uses, plants, water features, waste and water management systems, and so on, that are best suited to the niches available.

In your Zone 00 'personal permaculture plan' you can adapt this tool as a way to look at your own life as a whole. On a non-physical level, when considering your lifestyle, Zones 1 and 2 can be seen as the areas of your life into which you put most energy (i.e. homelife, work, studies, etc) and which therefore hopefully are most productive for you – if they are not it is time for some redesign of your life! Sectors can be seen as the areas where you have different types of energy coming in from the outside, which might be information, skills, money or friendship, inspiration or encouragement. Slopes can be seen as your motivations, with positive motivations being like a sunny or down-hill slope, helping you to move forward. Resistances, blockages and ruts in your life can be like up-hill slopes and dark or sunken areas – which can be made more productive through careful design.

Thinking about your life in this way, doing your own 'personal permaculture plan' for Zone 00, and applying permaculture design principles to the flows of energy, patterns and different zones of your life can be incredibly useful, enjoyable and productive.

Permaculture Techniques

Mulching is a key technique used in many permaculture systems, because it has so many benefits. Mulch is usually a thick layer of organic material over the soil – newspaper or cardboard is often used as a bottom layer, with several layers of organic materials on top. Black plastic (not my favorite) and old (organic i.e. wool) carpet are also sometimes used. In very dry areas rock mulches can also be effective.

a) Mulch is usually used:
- around plants, newly planted trees and trees that are already established to create good soil conditions for plant growth including reduced competition;
- to kill off weeds and prepare undug ground, and then plant new seedlings and trees into or through the mulch.

b) Mulching is very multi-functional as it:
- protects the soil from excessive heat, drying, cold, wind and rain;
- keeps the soil cool and moist in summer, and warm in winter;
- prevents and discourages unwanted plants from competing with those that have been planted - which is particularly important for young trees;
- adds to the fertility of the soil by providing an ideal home below the mulch for micro-organism, bacteria and worms to break down organic matter, thereby helping the soil to develop and release its own natural fertility without digging.

As a practical example, ideally mulch should be spread up to a metre around newly planted trees, say 5-10cm deep, leaving about 5-10cm around the trunk of the tree. In its early years this will assist the young tree and accelerate its healthy growth by a) creating excellent soil conditions for young roots to grow into, b) preventing competition for nutrients other plants in the mulched area, and c) making more nutrients available as the mulch breaks down.

In most climates ground cover plants can be used to create *a living mulch*. The general intention is to cover every area of soil, either with plants or with mulch. If you compare mulched soil with the soil in a non-organic arable field, the former is teeming with the life that allows it to build and release its fertility, while the latter is a largely dead soil which requires significant inputs to allow crops to be grown commercially.

Stacking is permaculture principle which is particularly well demonstrated within the forest garden concept and is illustrated in the forest garden diagrams in this section. Stacking involves using vertical space to its full extent, so that every level of the garden, from ground to canopy, are productive. Time Stacking is also used to plan for a harvest throughout the year – both these elements of stacking are indicated in the table of potential forest garden species in Appendix 3. Forest gardening and agroforestry are both examples of using stacking as a basic strategy, as explained in the following pages.

Establishing an *All-Year Salad Beds* and herb beds is a great project to start a permaculture garden or a forest garden. With a location and basic layout established, start with winter salads, then work on the spring and early summer salads. It is also possible to add fungi into your system, such as shitake mushrooms. (See forest garden table for suggested plant species).

Forest Gardening

The magic of the forest garden concept (sometimes called food forest, or edible landscape) is that it brings together so many other aspects of permaculture. One of your main design objectives for a home garden, community garden or small-holding might be to create a really good forest garden system. This involves the creation of a productive and stable, multi-layered 'miniforest' system, that is packed full of all sorts of food producing or otherwise useful plants, shrubs and trees. This is all rooted in an understanding of forest ecology, so it works with the different layers of a forest system, placing together plants that benefit each other. The forest garden is one of the most widely used ideas in permaculture because it's simple and effective, aiming to create and use up to seven layers in a garden or growing system – these are:

1. Canopy e.g. main fruit, timber and nut trees
2. Understorey / smaller trees (often shade tolerant) e.g. hazel/filberts, edible crab apple
3. Shrubs e.g. fruit bushes, mulch plants
4. Herbaceous: green veg, herbs, etc.
5. Ground cover e.g strawberries, herbs, greens, squash, etc.
6. Roots e.g. garlics, Jerusalem artichokes, main root crops, etc.
7. Climbers: vines, Siberian kiwi, thornless blackberry, nasturtium, runner bean, etc.
8. Fungi/Mycelium layer: for its activity below the surface and crops above.

The following diagrams and Appendix 3's table of example plants provide practical information on some of the many plants that can be used in these different layers (excluding the fungi layer). The aim is to make every layer productive and useful, and to create numerous beneficial relationships amongst plants and creatures within and between each layer.

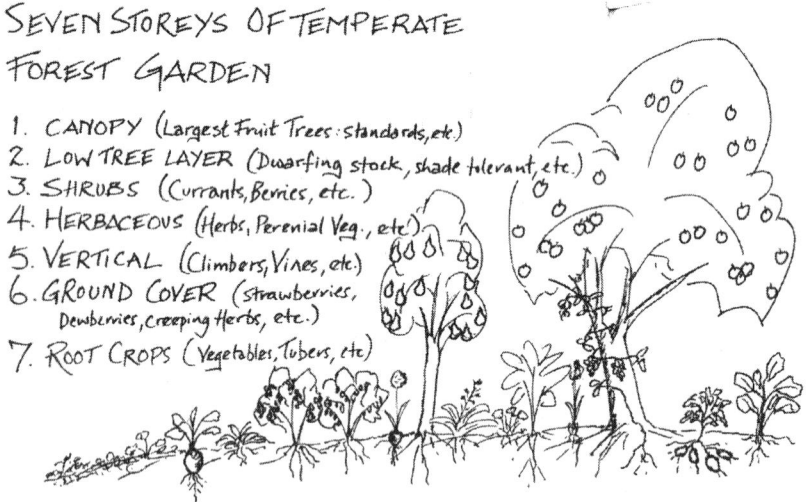

Seven Storeys Of Temperate Forest Garden

1. CANOPY (Largest Fruit Trees: standards, etc.)
2. LOW TREE LAYER (Dwarfing stock, shade tolerant, etc.)
3. SHRUBS (Currants, Berries, etc.)
4. HERBACEOUS (Herbs, Perenial Veg., etc.)
5. VERTICAL (Climbers, Vines, etc.)
6. GROUND COVER (strawberries, Dewberries, creeping Herbs, etc.)
7. ROOT CROPS (Vegetables, Tubers, etc)

The Forest Garden mimics the natural, therefore sustainable, forest ecosystem. It requires minimum maintenance, and it maximizes output, because it uses plants that naturally benefit each other – companion plants & 'guilds'.

"Diversity is the keynote of the forest garden concept, but it must be an ordered diversity, governed by the principles and laws of plant symbiosis; all plants must be compatible with each other. Most forest gardens are designed primarily to meet the needs of the cultivators and their families for food, fuel, fibres, timber and other necessities, but some can also include a cash component. The forest garden is the most productive of all forms of land use... [It] is far more than a system for supplying mankind's material needs. It is a way of life that also supplies people's spiritual needs by its beauty and the wealth of wildlife it attracts."

Robert Hart, the 'inventor' of forest gardening in Britain, from *Forest Gardening*, by Robert Hart, Green Books, Hartland, 1991.

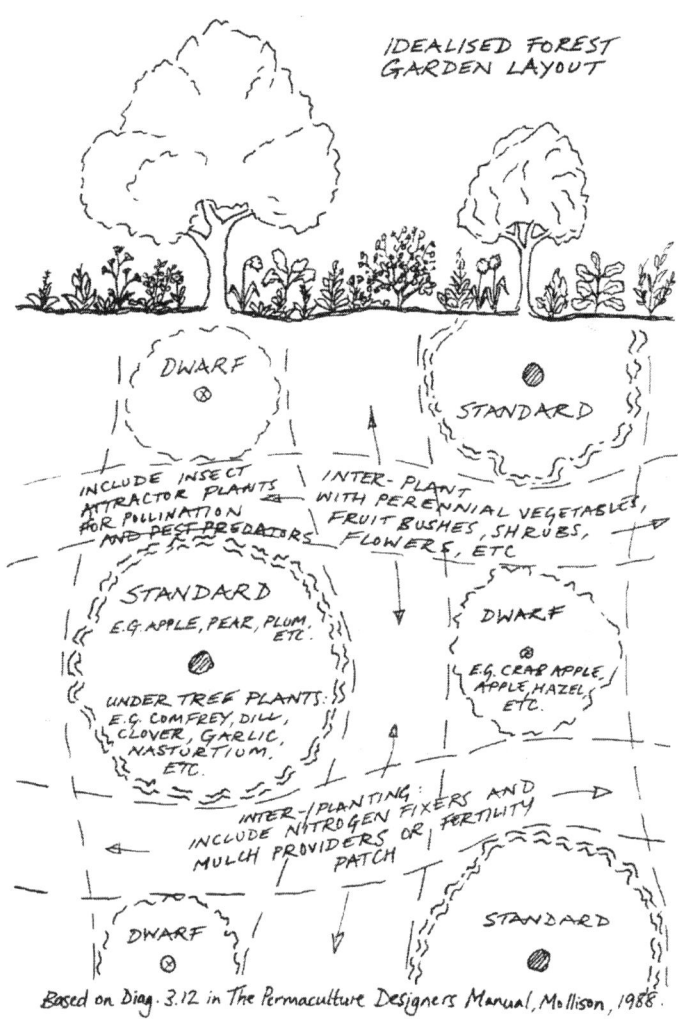

Based on Diag. 3.12 in *The Permaculture Designers Manual*, Mollison, 1988.

The leading British permaculture designer, teacher and author Patrick Whitefield preferred the term 'woodland garden', however, Patrick also felt that because the term 'forest garden' has become widely used it is easier to stick with that, hence the title of his excellent book: *How To Make A Forest Garden* (Permanent Publications, 1996).

... herbs and perennial vegetables are quite happy to look after themselves. They need little or no watering or composting, because their deep roots draw up water and minerals from the subsoil, for the benefit of themselves and each other, and they don't even need weeding or hoeing, as they quickly spread over the whole surface of the soil, suppressing all competitors, while their intricate tangle of roots maintain a porous soil-structure.

Robert Hart, from *The Forest Garden*, Inst. for Social Inventions, Third Edition, 1992.

In warmer climates and developing countries forest gardening is particularly effective and often familiar e.g. in Kenya, the Carribbean, etc. In severe situations, a forest garden can protect sensitive plants from intensive sun and wind, prevent soil erosion, promote water retention, help build-up of available groundwater, increase fertility and also provide many crops of course.

Forest gardens can usually be planted even in very marginal sites or regions – for example according to Bill Millison there are at least 30 food producing species of tree that grow in a desert situation. But the key point is that in most climatic conditions and in most soil types a well designed forest garden will bring good results - in difficult conditions it may take more work to establish, but also in those difficult conditions it may also bring the greatest benefits in the medium or longer term.

The best new forest garden resources are those produced by Martin Crawford of the Agroforestry Research Trust – the book *Creating a Forest Garden* (2010) and the DVD *A Year in a Forest Garden* (2010) are excellent. Through permaculture networks and contacts you will be able to source a range of other DVDs and online information to help you learn about forest gardening, including the excellent *Forest Gardening* DVD which features Robert Hart amongst others. This provides a wealth of inspiration on growing foods to eat both raw and cooked, with Michael and Julia Guerra being a fantastic example of the productivity that can be achieved with just a small garden. It also features Ken Fern of Plants for a Future, and includes a great deal of useful information on plants and the design of forest garden systems. Other excellent DVD's are *The Global Gardener, In Grave Danger of Falling Food*, and *The Forest Garden Year*. New DVD's and online films are emerging all the time – Geoff Lawton is one of those that is particularly productive in this area, providing outstanding information on warmer climate forest gardening.

Agroforestry simplifies forest garden thinking to use 3 or 4 layers, applying it on a larger and often commercial scale. It can involve a variety of techniques.

One approach is to model forest systems and use a diversity of plants around several key crops, which in a tropical climate might include bananas, papaya and cacao – cacao (the basic ingredient of chocolate) for example has to grow in shade, so is always grown as an understorey to other taller, shade producing trees.

Another agroforestry system is alley cropping, or inter-cropping, which involves planting a) rows of trees, with a mix of varieties and functions (e.g. fruit, timber, fertility crops, and/or nitrogen fixers), with b) productive / useful bushes underneath (e.g. fruit, nitrogen fixers), and then a gap between these rows where c) more traditional vegetable or arable crops are planted.

In many situations a well-designed agroforestry system is almost certainly the single most sustainable form of broad-scale productive land management because it harnesses CO_2 and raises soil fertility. This approach to land management is massively underused in the west because farms are designed to fit the machinery and an industrial, rather than a sustainable, approach to food production – although it is now being experimented with commercially. Agroforestry can easily be integrated into large scale food production systems – even if it only starts by taking up 5-10% of a farm. Agroforestry and forest gardening are seen by many as the most practical solution to sustainable food production in many of the ecologically degraded and desertified regions of the world and quite possibly the only practical solution - both in terms of ecological regeneration and sustained productivity. They are both productive and regenerative. They are also entirely appropriate for much more typical, average or highly productive soils and climates.

Regenerative Agriculture and **Whole Farm Systems** provide an ideal scale for the design and implementation of permaculture solutions. Reading Bill Mollison's *Introduction to Permaculture*, or the *Permaculture Designer's Manual* will show the application of integrated design of sustainable solutions at this **broadscale solutions** level – which is equally relevant for whole neighbourhoods, schools and their grounds, and other settlements and institutions. This is the scale Bill Mollison saw permaculture as most vital, because it is the scale at which modern agriculture is most destructive. There is increasing need to develop broad-scale permaculture farms, to put farmers through permaculture training, or to put peramculturalists through mainstream agricultural or horticultural training, so that people can work in agriculture and influence it from the inside, by working with the current nature of the agriculture industry, and gradually transforming it from within. The film *Inhabit* is a great illustration of what is possible.

In recent years **Regenerative Agriculture** (RegenAg), Holistic Management, Pasture Cropping and Polyface Farming have all become familiar, respected and influential terms at this broadscale level - mainly what is considered Zone 3 in permaculture. *Their focus is on developing regenerative processes through establishing ecologically beneficial relationships between soil, grazing and pasture.*

Useful Plants and Plant Typologies

Perennials, Self-Seeders, Companions and Guilds

Useful plants, like perennials, self-seeders and nitrogen fixers, are a vital part of permaculture – once started, unlike annual crops, they require little or no work to produce a harvest or fulfill various functions. Perennials include trees, shrubs and bushes, as well as perennial vegetables and herbs. Perennial greens are particularly valuable for providing high mineral and nutrient levels which are much closer to natural wild foods than manipulated annual vegetable strains. Using such plants within a forest garden shows how a low maintenance food producing system can be designed with perennials, self-seeders, companions and guilds (see below) of all types forming the foundations of that system.

The permaculture movement in general and the Agroforestry Research Trust and Plants For A Future projects in particular (see later section) have created a huge resource of useful information on all these kinds of plants, and the many uses they have – a resource that is easily accessible via books and the internet. Some examples of these useful plants are:

Cut'n'come again plants grow more when some of their leaves are harvested (e.g. chives, corn salad, rocket, spinach, pak choi, mizuna, radish, rape leaf, cabbage, land cress, leaf celery, lemon balm, red-leaved chicory, mint, parsley, coriander, endive, claytonia, purslane, etc.).

Pick'n'pluck vegetables give a harvest over a long period of time and include spinach beet, Swiss chard, sorrel, perennial broccoli, watercress, fennel, seakale, tree onions, Welsh onions and everlasting onions, garlic, horseradish, broad beans, courgette, angelica, lovage, sweet cicely, and so on.

Companion plants are plants that grow well together. Examples of good companions are tomatoes and marigolds.

Nitrogen Fixers and Fertility Plants, including mineral accumulators, have a particular role in creating excellent soil health and enabling fertility to be released to plant systems.

Guilds take these ideas further by creating groupings of 3 or more plants or other elements that work together, so that the whole is greater than the sum of its parts. The classic example of a guild is the native American combination of beans, maize and squash – a sacred combination called 'the Three Sisters'. The beans fix nitrogen and grow up the maize, while the squash produces a living mulch. They all produce a crop, whilst meeting each other's needs. A useful basic model of a guild is to include a) a nitrogen fixer or fertility plant, b) a vertical plant / element, and c) a ground cover plant / element – all productive in one or more ways.

In nutritional terms, a good balance of vitamins, minerals and food enzymes is a nutritional guild, because you obtain more nutritional value from foods which contain all of these. Having green leafy veg with either protein foods or starch foods is more of a 'companion food' than a nutritional guild. A guild is a consciously designed grouping that creates a combination and a whole effect that is greater and more positive than just the sum of its parts. It's like multiplying a group of numbers together, rather than adding them.

FLOWERING PLANTS, AND THE ROLE OF FLOWERS AND BEES

Flowers are particularly important in creating permaculture gardens and systems, and have many uses.

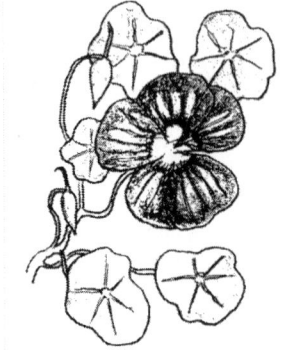

a) Flowers are vitally important for supporting bee / pollinator populations and a good insect habitat, which is essential for pollination and wildlife.

b) Beauty is a vitalising force –it's food for the soul!

c) Many flowers are also edible – such as mallow, nasturtiums, milkweeds, calendula, campanulas, yellow asphodel, chives, onions and the day lily, and make wonderful additions to salads.

Of course flowers are wonderful for bees, that have such a vital role in nature as a whole, and in human's food growing systems. So the role and placement of flowers needs careful thought within a permaculture or forest garden design. In the world as it is now, with bee populations devastated by agrochemicals, by insensitive and unwise exploitation of bees for commercial farming and commercial honey production, and by various factors which weaken their resistance to disease it could easily be argued that creating multifunctional food growing systems which are always designed to significant benefit bees is essential to humanity's long term ability to feed itself (see *The Barefoot Beekeeper* for more information).

WILD FOODS

Wild foods are the ultimate cheap, hugely nutritious food, as the excellent book *Food For Free* points out. It is important to know the poisonous wild plants, and to get to know the edible ones very well. Edible wild plants can be included in your garden, or harvested from around it. 'Wildcrafted' foods are often key ingredients in highly nutritious, high value superfoods, and are increasingly used in salads in some of the most expensive restaurants, with a number of leading Swiss and German chefs making a particular name for themselves in this area.

Wild greens (also often called wild-crafted foods) are generally recognized as being more mineral and nutrient rich than vegetables produced by conventional agriculture and horticulture. Franz Konz is well-known in the German natural health movement for promoting the health benefits of wild foods, whilst David Wolfe, Daniel Vitalis and others emphasize their benefits to the English-speaking raw world, with Rob Hull being particularly active in promoting the benefits of wild foods through the excellent *Funky Raw* magazine and website.

Many permaculturists and survival skills teachers are also great promoters and users of wild foods (both raw and cooked), with much of the greatest wild foods expertise lying in the wildness skills or survival skills movement (drawing particularly on the native American knowledge spread by Tom Brown Jnr in particular). Daniel Vitalis' talks on the subject of 'indigenous foods' (e.g. via Youtube) provide an excellent and entertaining explanation of how narrow our understanding of these issues generally is, and provides a sense of how removed we have become from working with nature, and its innate momentum towards creating health.

Even in towns and cities, by finding the surprising number of unpolluted and un-fouled places, wild foods can be a simple and nutritious addition to our diet. Dandelions, chickweed, ribbed plantain, lime tree leaves, Jack-by-the-Hedge (or hedge garlic), ransoms (or wild garlic), ground ivy (which has a 'love it or hate it' flavour), nettles, and then there's blackberries, chestnuts, hazelnuts and a variety of mushrooms (which need to be identified carefully of course) – all these can make their contribution. *Ginkgo biloba*, mulberries, medlars and other wonderful trees, whilst not wild, are also available in many public parks. And you can of course start to notice wild foods in your own garden, and stop seeing them as 'weeds'.

The importance of wild foods is that they've had no nurturing so they are strong and healthy as they are, where they are. They are native food plants. By eating them you are building that vital, vibrant, wild energy and strength into your body.

See *Food For Free*, Richard Mabey, or *Wild Food*, by Roger Phillips (Appendix 3); *Funky Raw* Magazine also includes regular articles on wild food plants.

Other Useful Plants

A range of useful plants will help increase the yield and health of the whole system, whether it is a forest garden or any other permaculture system:

- Nitrogen fixers: e.g. in temperate systems *Eleagnus*, clover, lucerne/alfalfa, beans, alder, black locust/false acacia, Siberian pea tree, etc. In sub-tropical/ Mediterranean climates: tagasaste, leucaena, albizia, beans, peas, lucernce/ alfalfa, etc.
- Mulch plants: e.g. reeds (*Phragmites australis/communis*), aromatic herbs to deter slugs (mints, tansy, balm, etc). Oak leaf mould is also a good slug deterrent.
- Pest repellents: e.g. onion/allium family (chive, garlic, etc.), marigolds, etc.
- Green manure/fertility patch: e.g. comfrey, clover, lucerne/alfalfa, buckwheat, chicory, dandelion, nettles, yarrow.
- Insect attractors for pollination: e.g. calendula, borage, chives, buddleia, etc.
- Host plants for predators of pest insects: e.g. chives, buckwheat.
- Species for pollination: e.g. crab apple.

The Design Process

As permaculture is a system of design, the design process is obviously important. There is no single 'right' way to do it. However, there are various tools and techniques, tricks processes and checklists that help to guide the design and implementation process. This section provides a basic, but very useful, introduction to the design process and the use of design tools within it, which can be applied to designing your diet, your lifestyle or your garden – or ideally all three. For a more in depth exploration and elucidation of these issues see the excellent book *Permaculture Design: a step by step guide* by Aranya (Permanent Publications, 2012).

Through studying permaculture on a course preferably, or from books and websites, and then applying it to your home and garden - or your health - you will develop a metaphorical 'Permaculture Tool Bag'. The point of using the tools described below is that they help to get more out of your design efforts and to do so easily – both during the design, as well as in the implementation and maintenance phases. Already by reading this far in the book you have gained a basic knowledge of your first tools in your permaculture tool bag:

- The permaculture ethics and principles.
- Zones, sectors and slope.
- Stacking.
- Mulching.
- Forest gardening and agroforestry.
- Perennials and self-seeders.
- Pick-n-pluck and cut-n-come-again salads.
- Companion planting and guilds.

A particularly important and useful tool is the OBREDIM checklist that guides you through the design process, as the following section explains.

The OBREDIM Design Process

OBREDIM is a fantastically useful tool for considering and addressing all sorts of situations, whether it's the design of a garden, your daily lifestyle, your health and diet, or your work and income. It provides you with a systematic process to survey the key issues, analyse the objectives and priorities, evaluate the resources available, and then to design and implement solutions, with its real power lying in its use in tandem with other permaculture principles, tools and techniques.

O - Objectives and Observation: for and of the site or situation, its uses and users, its characteristics and surroundings, the energy flowing through it, and so on. Get your objective clear first (although they can change with time), then initially *just stick to observation* (with eyes, ears and other senses), note down thoughts, and leave the designing until later.

B - Boundaries – record and map them. Walk the boundaries and look into the site, and away from it. Boundaries include time, money, knowledge, ethical and skills boundaries, for example, not just physical boundaries.

R - Resources and Research – identify, list and categorise the available biological, physical, energy, human and financial resources onsite and those available nearby. Research the site and location, the history, the possibilities, what's worked well and what's not worked in other designs.

E - Evaluate and Examine – of site data and other information; putting a 'value' to the things being considered in terms of priorities and their potential to help you achieve the objectives of your design. Considering what's been gathered from the O, B and R stages together for the first time.

D - Design – placing things together and creating the relationships between elements and flows that will enable you to achieve your design objectives e.g. up to 50%+ of food needs and a beautiful garden that's great for wildlife – using a range of design tools from your Permaculture Toolbag (see below).

I - Implement – including design phasing of implementation, and planning what resources you will need to use and when.

M - Monitor, Modify and Maintain – Get a feel for or look at how well your systems are working and make adjustments to either the system or your objectives – or both, as necessary.

OBREDIMET and SADIM are alternatives used by some, with the ET of the former covering Evaluate and Tweak (covered by the 3 M's used above), whilst the latter is a shorter summary of the design process: Survey, Analyse, Design, Implement, Monitor-Modify-Maintain.

Using OBREDIM with the 'Zone, Sector and Slope' tool gives you a basic framework for the design process and a structural overview of the design plan. Then within the design part of the OBREDIM process there is a wide range of design tools that you can pull out of your easily transportable 'permaculture tool bag'.

Your Permaculture Toolbag

Your permaculture toolbag is a weightless set of design and thinking tools and techniques that you can take anywhere, to assess sites, understand and define needs and relationships, and come up with creative and effective design solutions. Seven of the most useful tools which I always consider using within a design process from the start, are the following:

Multi-function (or the 'Three-Use Rule'): work out how all elements in a system can have at least three uses or benefits. A core principle in permaculture, this contains the essence of designing sustainable systems. So, a simple hedge can provide food, a wind break for plants and people, beauty, a wildlife habitat, produce bee food, and be a boundary marker and a barrier to keep larger animals out. A pond can provide food, relaxation and beauty, wildlife habitat and a home for slug-munching frogs, and if carefully placed it can reflect extra solar radiation into a conservatory or greenhouse in the winter. Similarly, a cycle path network can create a sustainable transport and wildlife corridor, be part of a public health and community art strategy, with sculptures lining the route, and be an education resource – it could also be planted to produce fruit for cyclists to snack on or harvest along the way!

Multi-Supply goes hand in hand with multi-function and aims to ensure that the needs of any element in the system are met by more than one supply. So a tree's need for water can be met by rain, mulching and ground-cover plants which reduce run-off and evaporation, and a landscaped water harvesting system to feed ground water supplies. Food supplies are met by a diverse range of plants so that many nutrients are supplied, harvests are available through much of the year and the system it has maximum resilience to pests through its diversity.

Input-Output Analysis involves looking at all the key elements of your system, site, home, self or lifestyle. In a garden this might include main-crop veg beds, pond, compost heap, all-year herb and salad garden, people, house, fruit trees and so on. You then list all the main inputs and outputs from each of those elements and then as much as possible locate each element so that every output from one element can automatically or easily become an input to at least one other element of the system i.e. kitchen scraps and garden waste go to the compost heap or help create mulch, and the compost or mulch feeds the soil, which feeds the veg and fruit plants, which feed the people, whose 'humanure' can be composted to feed the garden, and so on. Imagine doing this for Zone 0, inside your home too. This aims to ensure there is zero waste and to minimize the work involved in moving inputs and outputs around. It involves focusing on the connections and relationships between the elements, which is the essence of ecology.

Removal of Limiting Factors looks at the factors that are limiting the productivity, health or effectiveness of elements in the system – whether that's the garden, an organisation, or yourself. Then seeks strategies and actions to remove or reduce those limiting factors. So if lack of water is a limiting factor in a garden then improving water retention and collection, mulching and more efficient use of water are strategies to reduce that limiting factor. Limiting factors might include wind, shade, slope, soil quality, knowledge, practical skills, time, and where they cannot be removed or reduced, then adapting to the limiting factor is another option. Removal of Limiting Factors can always also be balanced by the tool of **Enhancing Positive Factors**, which seeks to identify the strengths and positives of a site or situation, to take further advantage of them to increase productivity, the range of yields, diversity and stability, and to reduce work inputs.

Wild design is another approach to design that uses processes which consciously utilise chance or creative chaos as a catalyst for ideas and inspiration – this can be a lot of fun. Wild design is then followed by a consideration or evaluation of what useful and creative ideas have appeared, and putting aside those that are not useful.

Thematic design analyses and/or designs by looking at one theme at a time, such as plants, water, energy, animals, structures or events/activities. For a person or lifestyle it might involve analyzing or design systems of work life, home life, leisure, diet, creativity and so on.

Visualisation techniques and Visioning can be used to imagine what your established permaculture system might look like ten years in the future, how to get there, and the practical first steps towards that vision ... a vision of a highly productive, healthy and beautiful garden, home, community or neighbourhood project ... or a vision of a highly productive, naturally healthy and beautiful you. Try it out.

YOUR HEALTH AND SUSTAINABILITY PATHWAY

So many design tools that can be used, whether your objective is health, sustainability or both. And the best way to learn how to use them is to do a permaculture design course. Although few permaculture courses yet address the design and creation of natural health in a genuinely open and ecological way, there is no limit to you applying what you learn in a design course to the subject of health creation, as well as to the more typical themes of food, garden, community and home. And as far as personal and community sustainability go there is no better source of learning and inspiration than a permaculture course.

Introduction to Permaculture (Bill Mollison, Tagari Press, 2000) is probably the best book for getting a feel for these things. Going on a course is even better and the best thing you can do for understanding how the various design methods and tools work in practice.

You can consult permaculture magazines and websites to find the exciting range of permaculture courses now on offer (particularly www.permaculture.org.uk, Permaculture Magazine, Permaculture Works). If you find you really enjoy it, you can then do a 2 year permaculture diploma, or study remotely via Gaia University (in English or Spanish). Joining local permaculture groups or networks and going on specialist courses are other excellent ways you can develop your knowledge and skills as you travel down your permacutlure pathway. Set some objectives along the way, for what you want to do or learn in the next year or two, but don't be too rigidly attached to them, because as you travel your path, your needs, interests and motivations may change, which may well alter your objectives.

GROWING AND BUYING FOODS TO COOK

It is far easier and better for the soil to grow foods that you can cook very simply (i.e. just cleaning them and then cooking them unprocessed with their skins, such as potatoes) than to even consider growing your own wheat / grains to make some kind of bread or pasta. How much work, machinery and energy is used to produce a loaf of bread, compared to a bowl of potatoes? Either on a local, organic or industrial scale? When you actually think about it this involves a huge amount of processing, energy, additional ingredients, baking equipment and infrastructure. Tubers also produce less mucus in the body than grains. I am not including much on this topic because there are plenty of excellent organic food and permaculture books to help you with both the growing techniques and types of plants to grow if you want to cook them.[89] And I am including it towards the end of this section as obviously the emphasis of this book is on raw foods.

However, it seems to me far healthier, easier and more multi-functional to grow starchy tubers and roots than it is to grow, harvest, process and cook grains, particularly wheat. It is also far better to use fresh produce than tinned or packaged produce – the energy used to get tinned peas to the table is estimated to be ten times greater than that for fresh peas for example.

Squashes and many other starchy vegetables can be eaten raw or cooked. Chilacoyote is a fun plant to grow – it's a marrow family plant (Curcubita), is very productive, and can store for years. The fruit can be baked, boiled or steamed. You will need space for it to grow though, as it's shoots will ramble off for many metres! Even with a small garden, on a hygienist type diet (i.e. without meat, grains or dairy) of around 70% raw or more, you can achieve extremely high levels of self-reliance in your food production, even in temperate climates, growing root vegetables, squash, beans and even grains in an intensive and diverse multi-layered forest garden/ permaculture system. This will have fantastic ripple effects.

If you are really being serious about changing from food habits that are environmentally damaging switch to growing your own root vegetables to cook, and leave the grain products behind. If you insist on growing some grains then millet, quinoa and amaranth are good to try in the right climates - and are good to sprout, which is the easiest form of grain processing. English grown quinoa can now also be bought. Wheat can also be easily sprouted, and this uses massively less energy than other wheat processing to make bread. Oats are a natural grain for more northerly climates, and can simply be eaten rolled or sprouted.

Useful Resources

In particular the following books will help to expand on the topics outlined in this section:
- *Introduction to Permaculture* (by Bill Mollison et al);
- *Forest Gardening* (by Robert Hart);
- *Creating a Forest Garden* (by Martin Crawford)
- *The Permaculture Garden* (by Graham Bell);
- *The Earth Care Manual, How To Make A Forest Garden* and *Permaculture In A Nutshell* (by Patrick Whitefield);
- *Permaculture: Principles and Pathways Beyond Sustainability* (by David Holmgren);
- *Permaculture Design: a step by step guide* (by Aranya)

Note: all above available from the Green Shopping Catalogue or online at: www.green-shopping.co.uk

---

[89] e.g. *The Permaculture Garden* by Graham Bell, *Plants for a Future* by Ken Fern, and Patrick Whitefield's books – see Appendices for full details – all available from www.green-shopping.co.uk

If you read and use any three or more of these books you'll be well on your way. *Permaculture Magazine*, published internationally by Permanent Publications, and the associated website www.permaculture.co.uk are superb sources of information for establishing forest gardens, agroforestry and permaculture systems in any climate. *The Permaculture Activist* (USA) is a great voice for a more theoretical view of permaculture, as well as for projects and courses in north America. The best 3 things to do are a) to buy yourself a copy of one of these magazines, b) join the Permaculture Association (if you are in Britain), and in particular c) go to the courses section at the back or on the Permaculture Association website (www.permaculture.org.uk) and book yourself on a permaculture course right away. Simple!

Appendix 3 contains a more extensive list of books and sources of information.

PART 8: THERE'S LOTS OF INFORMATION & INSPIRATION OUT THERE

SECTION ONE: LIFESTYLES, LANDSCAPES AND PHILOSOPHIES OF LIVING

This section of the book includes contributions from inspiring, wise and experienced friends and contacts with active roles in the natural health and raw food movements, and is dedicated to Robert Hart, who died in 2000, age 86, and who's contribution opens this section of the book.

Although I only knew him in his later years, Robert Hart was a particular inspiration. In effect Robert 'invented' the concept of the forest garden, at least for western gardeners and horticulturalists, with his work recognised with an award from the Institute for Social Inventions. He was particularly inspired by Mahatma Gandhi, and worked for Reuters putting out Gandhi's weekly newsletters to the world through the Reuters news and information networks. Robert returned to the land as a smaller farmer, caring for his mother and his brother, and lived simply for many years, eventually developing the most complete and well established forest garden in Britain at his home in Shropshire. He inspired, encouraged and informed literally thousands of people who came to visit his garden and read his many books and articles. He strongly encouraged me to write this book, and as my maternal family name is Hart, I felt a particular connection with Robert.

The development of both Agroforestry Research Trust and the Plants for a Future project which are mentioned in this section, have been natural evolutions which follow on from Robert's inspiring work, improving it as they go, and also driven forward by the commitment of a next wave of passionate and fantastically knowledgeable individuals.

THE FOREST GARDEN DIET, LIFESTYLE AND PHILOSOPHY, BY ROBERT A DE J HART

When I first took over my small organic farm on Wenlock Edge in Shropshire I had two main enterprises:

1. Rearing dairy heifers for sale after calving.
2. The provision of nourishing food for my invalid mother, brother and myself.

Over the years I have learnt a great deal, by study and experience, about farming, gardening, human health and nutrition.

The ideal diet for positive health, I am convinced, consists mainly of fresh or sun-dried fruit, vegetables and herbs, consumed 70% raw. Fruit sugars feed the brain and energise the body, while chlorophyll, the green pigment which has a chemical constitution similar to that of human blood, uses solar radiation to create carbohydrates and this is the basis of physical life.

In striving to develop a system of land-working which could supply the core ingredients of such a diet throughout the year, in restricted areas and with minimum labour, I have discovered that the time-honoured system known as forest gardening or home gardening, which is practised in many countries, is the most effective, imitating, as it does, the natural forest. One of the basic dishes of the forest garden at Highwood Hill is the 'sallet', comprising a wide variety of fruit, vegetables, nuts and herbs, as consumed in the Great Age of Herbalism, in the 17th century. As the palate gets accustomed to the strong, vital flavours of raw plant foods, the more delicious and satisfying they become.

One ceases to crave for animal foods and cereals, which undoubtedly have a clogging and acidifying effect on the system and therefore, sooner or later, lead to degenerative disease. The 'fruit and greenery' diet is alkaline and eliminative and therefore maintains the free and sweet circulation of the blood and other bodily fluids, which is an outstanding feature of positive health. From painful experience, I learned that the provision of dairy products involves as much cruelty and slaughter as the provision of meat. In particular, the separation of the newborn calf from its mother, which is essential for milk production, is a traumatic experience for both cow and calf. Out of compassion, as well as for health reasons, I have been a vegan for some 15 years.

I also avoid gluten cereals – wheat, barley, oats, and rye – as gluten, which is a protein, undoubtedly has a clogging effect on the blood-stream, leading to a build-up of toxins. Favouring, as I do, minimum cooking, I avoid baked and fried foods; the only cooking I do is to lightly boil roots and certain other vegetables in spring water, which I thicken with maize flour, millet or gram (ground lentils). The forest garden diet is part of a compassionate, non-consumerist and sustainable lifestyle, which involves conservation of the environment and involves a sense of close communion with nature. If it were generally adopted, disease and malnutrition throughout the world could be reduced to a minimum.

If forest gardening and agroforestry become much more widespread, both in 'developed' and 'developing' nations, then the 'bioregions', which are the life-supporting areas surrounding residential centres, can be developed in such a way as to ensure regular supplies of fresh plant foods, timbers, fibres and other useful materials for everyone – town dwellers and countryfolk alike. This can be the basis on which a diverse, sophisticated, bountiful, beautiful, sustainable and positively healthy 21st century culture can thrive.

Robert Hart, 1913-2000.

INDOOR GARDENING AND LIVING FOODS, BY ELAINE BRUCE

This section is compiled and edited from an article by Elaine Bruce in Permaculture Magazine No.9, and an interview with Elaine in The FRESH Network News, Feb - April, 1999.

Through using windowsills and shelves, and all sorts of indoor spaces, to grow many plants, indoor gardening is an important part of a 'Living Foods Lifestyle' which aims for 'super nutrition' by supplying fresh organic foods, with the extra dimension of enzyme rich and chlorophyll rich foods. This is a very powerful way of repairing cells and boosting immunity.

To supply these powerful healing and cleansing foods with relatively little effort in particular involves growing sprouted seeds (e.g. alfalfa, green lentils, mung beans, chick peas, radish, quinoa, etc.) and 'indoor greens' (young shoots, such as sunflower, radish or buckwheat) which can be eaten in salads, in cold green energy soups or juiced. Sprouting in jars and trays can supply large quantities of top quality organic foods, at a low cost – especially if you buy in bulk, perhaps with friends, from a wholefood co-op.

Most seeds just need soaking over-night and rinsing daily. Depending on the temperature and type, your delicious sprouts will be ready in two, three or four days – voila! Green lentils, chick peas and quinoa are quick sprouters; mung beans and alfalfa take a day or so more.

Chlorophyll is concentrated in the leaves of 'indoor greens' and wheat grass and is especially powerful in detoxifying the body and rebuilding living tissue. Its chemical structure is almost identical to that of haemoglobin in blood. Wheat-grass juice (i.e. the juice from sprouted wheat grain, grown in a tray on a thin bed of compost) is the ultimate chlorophyll provider. The powerful green juice is squeezed out of the grass using special manual or electric juicers. [90]

Dr. Ann Wigmore, who established the Living Foods Programme, was a lively, dynamic person. Shining with health and vitality, she was totally focused on her teaching - she and her associates have taught many people around the world.

Perhaps inspired by one of the many excellent books on the subject, the normal route to living foods is via a course, which is an enjoyable blend of practical hands-on sessions and theory. They start with the basics of growing a complete range of sprouted seeds and year-round indoor greens. Many recipes and techniques are demonstrated on a course in order to give all the information needed to establish a Living Foods kitchen. The processes of food fermentation and dehydration are explained and freshly made dishes are served immediately with an abundance of fresh organic produce. Emphasis is placed on the uses of chlorophyll as the most efficient and inexpensive way to maintain health and vitality. The courses also look at detoxification and healing, and how to manage the transition process to Living Foods.

A Living Foods kitchen with its indoor garden takes no more daily time than cooker or freezer based routines; more time is spent on washing salads and scrubbing veggies and on daily care of indoor greens and sprouts. This is more than offset by time saved on shopping, storage, preparing/cooking and washing up.

In Elaine's Living Foods kitchen you will find...

INDOOR GREENS grown in trays of compost. The seeds of sunflower and buckwheat are popular; radish and even fenugreek can also be used. These are soaked, allowed to germinate, and then spread to grow on compost laid thinly on a tray. They are kept in the dark (damp but not wet) for a few days and then put in window racks to green for a few days. They are then ready to be cut near the base to be eaten fresh and vital in salads or juiced. Indoor greens provide cheap, high-quality fresh organic greens, full of natural nutrients, throughout the year.

WHEATGRASS is grown in the same way. After some days when it has grown to perhaps six inches, it is cut and juiced to give a daily dose of healthy vitamins, especially the anti-oxidants, and plant enzymes. Fresh chlorophyll both nourishes and cleanses the tissues and helps to protect against radiation and chemical pollution. Hand powered wheatgrass juicers are very affordable for those that want to avoid electrical equipment.

SPROUTED SEEDS are kept in jars, with plenty of room for air and growth. This can include crunchy sprouts like chickpeas and lentils, soft sweet ones like aduki and mung, hot or spicy ones like mustard and fenugreek, and the best one of all for vitamins – alfalfa. Sprouted seeds and nuts are used both as they are and in recipes for raw patés, humous, tabbouleh, seed loaves and

---

[90] Steve's note: It is also possible to combine the Living Foods and 'Food For Free' concepts by using areas of uncut grass and / or a patch of nettles as a green juice factory.

nut cheese. Some are made into dehydrator crisps and cookies, both sweet and savoury – these are particularly good for those in transition to a raw living foods diet.

SURPLUS PRODUCE from the garden can be dehydrated and stored. Sliced dried tomatoes and onions make wonderful flavourings. Raspberries, sliced peaches, apricots, and wild blackberries can be reconstituted in a little spring water for fruit salads in winter.

JUICERS are used daily to make green drinks and vegetable and fruit juices.

FERMENTED FOODS are also an important item: sauerkraut, rejuvelac (fermented wheat grain soaked in water), and seed cheeses.

A few things are very gently cooked. Millet, sometimes known as 'the Queen of grains' is a seed used as an alkalinising grain substitute, and is very useful for those in transition. It only needs a short spell of low heat to soften the seed coats. Sometimes a potassium broth is used to regulate the acid/alkaline balance of the body.

Elaine has been practising and teaching the Living Foods Programme for many years. Taught by Dr. Ann Wigmore, in Boston in 1980, she joined her staff at the Puerto Rico Clinic for a time in 1992. She has trained and studied intensively in Naturopathy and Homeopathy. Elaine runs courses in Shropshire (UK) on the complete Living Foods lifestyle, and has been on a Living Foods diet for eighteen years, 100% raw for most of that time. She is also a trained permaculture designer. Elaine's book Living Foods for Radiant Health is widely available and her website at www.livingfoods.co.uk *also includes a DVD and CD, and course details. Other specialist books on Living Foods and sprouting, as well as wheatgrass juicers and other juicers are available from Elaine or from Hippocrates Health Institute in the USA – see Appendix 3.*

PARADISE GARDENING, BY JOE HOLLIS

The following has been distilled and edited from a slightly longer article by Joe Hollis

Paradise is, first of all, a garden, where everything we need is there for the taking. Paradise Gardening is a way of life which maintains the garden, and which is also maintained by that garden; a way of living that uses a small fraction of the available energy, whilst serving the continued survival and functioning of the garden ecosystem.

Everything needed to be completely human is available in the environment – the garden and the neighbourhood – it must be because 'human-ness' is a creation of the environment. You and I are recent manifestations of a co-evolution between our genes and all the other genes 'out there' – a co-evolution that began with the start of life on earth. So when we live in Paradise Garden we are specialists of working with nature to help create and sustain diversity.

In the modern world clearly there can be no going back to foraging. However, there can be going forward to Paradise Gardening – which can be described as 'intensified foraging'. This is a move from massive agricultural manipulation of ecosystems, to more subtle transformation of ecosystems. This involves the alteration of selected components of the natural system rather than its wholesale replacement. It is a method of cultivation which places certain preferred species in particularly suitable ecological niches, to simulate the structures and dynamics of the natural ecosystem. This is based on the realisation that "many 'non-agricultural' people were in fact engaged in intensive and sophisticated plant exploitation, previously unrecognized because their plant management practices did not fit into our idea of agriculture." (Harris, Ed. *From Foraging To Farming*)

On this path, our goal is to 'naturalise' ourselves in the environment, changing ourselves and the environment to an ecological 'fit' that suits both. What we need *now* is a process that leads us to that garden, that is justified in its own terms. Seeking the 'ideal' Paradise Garden will only perpetuate the same old patterns of selling out the present for some imagined better future.

We are widespread and greedy; evolution and natural succession indicate that eventually the 'competitive advantage' will pass to those who practice permanence, rootedness, slow growth and steady accumulation, with vertical expansion of the human spirit into uncharted or long-forgotten realms. Paradise Gardening involves re-attaching our life-support systems to the natural world of the garden and the neighbourhood. This is a gradual process requiring a deep analysis of our needs and expenditures (of physical, emotional and mental energy, as well as of money).

The Tao Te Ching says: '*The country over the border may be so close that one could hear the cocks crowing and the dogs barking in it, but the people would grow old and die without ever once troubling to go there.*'

Satisfaction of needs by the consumer system normally declines rapidly after the purchase. Needs met through our interaction with nature are more deeply met, with wonderful surprises along the way – as most people who have made anything 'from scratch' will know. What seldom occurs to us is that an entire life can be lived in this way; through a re-integration of needs.

Food, exercise, healing, entertainment, learning, creativity, spiritual inspiration – all these needs can be met by the paradise garden at the same time. This begins with both the present vegetation and the potential 'natural' vegetation, and to this are added species from similar ecosystems worldwide, with slight habitat enhancements. This brings about possibilities for new species; a 'cornucopia' never available to previous generations. 'Planned biotic enrichment' is within our power – to not only hold down the rate of species extinction but to reverse it, through 'species packing' which creates assorted equilibria that exceed any occurring in nature. This game of life involves creating new (biotic) communities and ecosystem transformations, which offer creative work with huge benefits to people, place and planet. We live within a narrow 'window of opportunity' – and we cannot put off our choice for any more lifetimes. A revolutionary shift is needed. We have little time to achieve this transition – before long the environment will be too degraded, the soils too depleted, the waters too polluted, the resources lost, with too many species extinct, and a human population that has increased massively. The paper tiger of more trade and economic growth just cannot deliver in to the future.

We all have two hands, one lifetime, twenty-four hours a day. This democratic factor means we can all help create a Paradise with relevance for all. Paradise Gardening at the personal, communal / neighbourhood and social level is vastly more meaningful than any bio-dome experiment to a world in need of examples that show a 'better' way – a sustainable, democratic and life-enhancing way.

For more information about Paradise Gardening contact:

Joe Hollis, Mountain Gardens, 546 Shuford Creek Road, Burnsville, NC 28714. USA. http://www.mountaingardensherbs.com/ - email: joehollis@excite.com
Joe Hollis also co-ordinates the Permaculture Seed and Plant Exchange.

FREE AND NATURAL LIFE: ON THE TRAIL OF SIMPLICITY AND LOVE, BY SIBILA

(Translated and edited from Spanish by Steve Charter)

Listening to Instinct

My single purpose is to bring myself closer and closer to oneness with the Whole. *I am ONE with the WHOLE, the Universe is in me and I in it because we are the same...* My desire is to live in this feeling constantly, with constant awareness and fullness... And it turns out that the most direct way to connect with the whole is to connect with *myself*, with my essence.

To be faithful to this path my existence cannot be based on external things, other people, books and so on. They serve me sometimes as ideas to consider and as a way to explore my own experience, until I am able to see or feel if their truth runs through my veins, in a way that makes me to want to welcome it into my life.

Initially, this way of being came to me from within, and I did not question my apparent inability to follow idols, gurus or teachers, whether in music, visual arts, literature, nutrition, clothes or spirituality. I liked to read everything and from this I gained and welcomed many things - but nothing tied me to one particular path. An enjoyment of solitude, alongside my lack of self-understanding and my lack of knowing how to feel and to live life (in family situations and in society), led me to what my parents called 'living in a turtle's shell'.

From adolescence, a newspaper which questioned everything helped me investigate my feelings about issues and explore them in a deep sense. I began to listen to my instinct and little by little everything was changing within me. To avoid suffering in vain, I was valuing things differently, and in this way I came to learn detachment. Detachment towards the family, friends, sex, possessions - and even food and the culture I lived in. When you become more and more intimate with yourself, relying on yourself more and more and, connecting more to Nature, little by little, your life becomes simpler and less confused. With that simplicity, for me, there is now no place for cooking and everything it entails.

If I now think about buying food and detergent, the cleaning of a conventional house, cooking, mopping, preparing the table, feeding the children at set times, and so on, it's very clear. Heavens! What a pile of work!

When I truly see and feel the energy of things, I discover that when I eat something the energy and feeling of it merges with me. If I eat something with a low vibration, then my body requires concerted efforts to turn it into life, a higher vibration, which drains me of certain minerals and vital energy. My body says to me: I want simplicity!

There are many ways and/or reasons to arrive at an eat more raw lifestyle. It can be a good theoretical book, a desperate search to recover lost health, or a cast-iron desire not to consume anything that entails materialism. Or simply you can listen to your instinct.

Taking myself to live in nature without a house with heating, was a decisive act for me. I connected so much with myself that simplicity just appeared and the chains were broken. The more I removed myself the more centered I have been and the more connected to Nature – and the less I needed anything cooked. Here, in my home, in the countryside, the choice is easy: Why put a lower vibration into my body when my children and I can eat something made by nature to be beneficial to us. If you begin to listen and to allow yourself to be yourself, the fullness of life will flow into you. Although in the beginning you may shed some tears for people, customs, or things that will disappear from your life, that is only temporary. It will be fully replaced by an eternal fullness born of simplicity and freedom, and of a love of the connection with Nature and the Universe, with yourself and with the Whole... Then many other things will follow one-by-one, little-by-little, without pain, making clear to you that all these aspects comprise just one single law – the Law of Universal Energy and Love.

For me raw food is not only a question of health, it is much more than that. It is a powerful questioning, and is a spiritual path as well as one that brings a more simple life, and frees my essence, in search of my original self. The path of that search is one of sincerity and purity, allowing me to be myself, through instinct. Listening to my instinct I am following my own path. I am my own guru and teacher. She or he is wise who faithfully only obeys universal laws and thereby benefits from them. And, if sometimes I do not follow them, it is not from ignorance of that law, but by being conscious of my emotional and psychic limitations, which are not instinctive. In these cases, I let it be, and my inner wisdom allows me to be less chained in my life every day.

Looking For Simplicity

Now I have only the memory of a life when I worked seven hours away from home, studied at university, had numerous possessions and clothes that all needed work to support (to buy them and look after them), as well as cleaning. Almost every day I spent two to four hours in the kitchen, making elaborate dishes, bread, yogurt, cheese, seitán, tofu, cakes and other complicated things. Dedicating so much time to all those things, I now ask myself where was there any space left for me? And I thank heavens I did not have a television! Now I see that my life was spiritually very poor; it was materialistic and superficial. Yes, I enjoyed doing all those things and some of those possessions but now, with the passage of the years, I have seen that they offer diversions but not a fullness or fulfillment in life, because they *are* diversions, born of a culture, not of the heart, the instinct, or nature... diversions that are great chains to our spirit. Although we learn to live with them, they do not stop being chains. I definitely prefer freedom - and freedom always comes from simplicity.

If I ever doubt whether I've done something by instinct or by culture, I ask myself how I would have acted 25, 30 or 50 centuries ago... then I always see the light. Through this light, I decide with consciousness, not through inertia. If I choose to go with my sense of how I would have acted centuries before, I find no benefits in what I was tied to before – and in this way I choose a new path, which is my own path.

If I choose to go with standard cultural norms, I find I am not taking responsibility for my own actions, including my unhealthy dependencies, habits and blockages. Then I remind myself that I am capable of anything and everything – I just have to know clearly what I want, allow time for this to happen and to trust. To trust Love and Universal Energy, which is to trust myself.

Nuria Aragon Castro, previously known as Sibila

The above is edited and translated from the introduction to Nuria/Sibila's first book: *Vida Libre y Natural: en el sendero de la sencillez y el amor* (Free and Natural Life: on the path of simplicity and love). See Appendix 3 for details of books (in Spanish), talks and art by Nuria Aragon Castro / Sibila, and visit *www.nuriaaragoncastro.com*

Nuria, a mother of two, is a powerful, loving inspiration to many people. She is an author, artist, speaker and a passionate advocate of home-education, natural health and a compassionate, cruelty-free way of life, having found her way through her own challenging experiments, explorations and experience in life. She has taken her beliefs and lifestyle to a variety of extremes as a process through which she has arrived at her truth – a truth which has relevance to anyone and everyone.

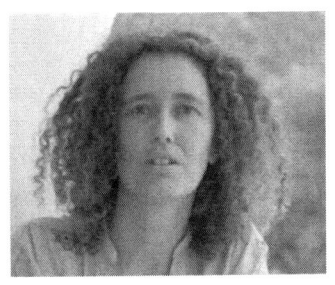

PLANTS FOR A FUTURE AND THE AGROFORESTRY RESEARCH TRUST

The *'Plants For A Future'* concept is highly relevant for linking excellent nutrition with food growing – it is that we can, with knowledge, meet all or most of our needs from plants and plant products – and that this a very positive move to take for people and planet.

Plants for a Future (PFAF - registered Charity Number 1057719) is a non-profit charitable education and research project, with demonstration sites and supplying information on a vast range of useful perennial plants that can be grown in a temperate climate. Their plants are grown with vegan organic methods. PFAF was established in 1989 at Penpol near Lostwithiel in Cornwall to grow and demonstrate the PFAF concept. Following years of research into plant uses, they have around 1,700 varieties of edible and otherwise useful plants growing at their sites. A degraded 25 acre field has been transformed into a lush woodland, and provides many needs such as food, wood, fibres and soap plants, and wonderful habitat. The PFAF online database includes around 7000 useful species, with printed information also available by post.

Please support *Plants For A Future* and help seed and spread the PFAF concept all around the world to every climate zone! For more information see: http://www.pfaf.org

The **Agroforestry Research Trust** is another hugely valuable and inspiring plant project (Charity No.1007440). Run by Martin Crawford and based in south Devon (UK), ART researches and demonstrates the viability of agroforestry in the temperate climate, with research and demonstration sites, through the provision of high quality information and through the sale of an excellent range of plants and seeds.

ART manages the 2 acre Schumacher Forest Garden Project on the Dartington estate, the 0.5acre companion tree experiment on land provided by the scientist James Lovelock, and a further 8 acres of trial grounds also on the Dartington Estate. The Forest Garden project aims to use 35,000 different plants to create a self-managing productive ecosystem using nitro-fixing plants and deep rooting dynamic accumulators to help maintain and improve the soil fertility.

The Trust provides fantastic information through its reports and Journal, as well as a superb range of plants and seeds, courses and guided tours. It's demonstration projects are the most sophisticated demonstration of the principles of stacking and plant diversity in the UK.

For courses, books, more information and to support Martin and ART's work contact: **Agroforestry Research Trust**, 46 Hunters Moon, Dartington, Devon. TQ9 6JT.
Website: www.agroforestry.co.uk, mail@agroforestry.co.uk

SECTION TWO: EXAMPLES OF MAJOR HEALING & PERSONAL CHANGE

JATINDA DANIELS: CURED SEVERE ARTHRITIS

"I was diagnosed with rheumatoid arthritis at the age of 16 and doctors said my future was bleak," says Jatinder, a healthy 45. "They said I could be in a wheelchair by the end of my teens, that I would be in varying degrees of constant pain for the rest of my life and, due to aggressive drugs, may not be able to have children. It was like a death sentence. "But look at me now! I'm a mum of three, perfectly mobile and free from the agony I endured for years. And it's all down to my raw food, low-toxin lifestyle."

Jatinder's teenage years in Nottingham were dogged with frustration and confusion over her stiffness and pain until, after endless tests, she was diagnosed. "I was healthy until 13 when I was vaccinated against rubella in school," Jatinder recalls. "My health deteriorated rapidly afterwards. Suddenly I couldn't do any sports at all. I was persistently tired and regularly in terrible pain. There were days when I couldn't walk, dress myself or bathe. Sometimes my jaw was so stiff I couldn't eat at all or just manage soup."

Jatinder went to hospital once a week for six months for injections into her joints yet the arthritis intensified and her knuckles and knees began to deform. She became suicidal. "The injections offered no immediate relief. I felt alone, angry and full of resentment. I was trying to do my A-levels but I couldn't even carry my own books. My condition worsened during the winter. The cold wind went straight to my bones and was agony. I became very depressed and often thought about throwing myself into the River Trent."

Despite being in constant pain, Jatinder was determined to live life to the full and at 21 went to London to study computing. "I needed a walking stick by the time I went to university but I refused to use one out of pride. I felt so vulnerable. I was adamant that I was going to be independent."

She explains: "The doctors had warned that I would have difficulty conceiving because of the drugs I'd been taking, so Raman was extra special. But caring for him was the biggest challenge I'd ever faced. "The normal duties that new mums take for granted like bathing their child was like climbing a mountain. But I had no choice but to cope."

Their second child Priyanka was born four years later and developed chronic eczema and asthma at eight weeks. The lack of sleep and stress that caused only made Jatinder's condition worse. She said: "I was beginning to think I couldn't go on. I couldn't see myself reaching my 40th birthday and if I'm honest part of me didn't want to if it meant living with constant pain. I believed it was only going to get worse."

It was during these dark times that Derek discovered the raw food way of life on the internet. He read claims that nature intended us to eat raw, whole food and that it is unnatural to consume cooked or processed foods. Jatinder explains: "Long-term consumption of processed food will lead to toxicity or toxaemia - when the body is overloaded with poisons. These harmful toxins are found all around us - in our environment, treated water, non-organic fruit and vegetables and cooked food. Raw foodists believe that major illnesses like cancer, diabetes and arthritis are often a result of toxaemia and can be prevented and greatly helped by a raw food way of life."

Jatinder says she realised the importance of food in relation to wellbeing years ago but the idea of eating only raw food seemed impossible. "I had stopped eating wheat years earlier noticing that wheat flour made my joints flare up and I had become vegan the previous year for similar reasons," she says. "I put the fact that I wasn't already in a wheelchair down to my healthy diet and generally positive mindset.

"I believed that food could have a miraculous effect on health, I just didn't believe I could take such drastic measures." When Jatinder conceived her youngest son Mohan, at the age of 37, she knew something had to be done to improve her health. So, at two months pregnant, she changed her diet to 100 per cent raw for one week. She says: "I had diarrhoea but felt the benefit and the pain reduced. "I went back to 50 per cent cooked until the following summer when the whole family began to detox."

The family moved to Spain four years ago where Jatinder is a raw food consultant. They live in beautiful whitewashed mountainside village on the Costa del Sol and the children attend the local school. "We wanted the children to grow up in a natural environment and I believe sunshine is another key to good health," she says.

And the family insist the raw food diet is fun and tasty. "Now the kids love it," Jatinder laughs. "There is so much variety. I make biscuits, crackers, sweets and some really tasty desserts. "Just like you learn how to cook, you can learn how to uncook. It is amazing what textures you can achieve by using a blender or the food you can create simply by dehydrating it. It may sound complicated but once you've got the hang of it, the preparation time is actually less. Friends who come around for lunch are amazed when I tell them what they are eating is in fact raw."

Jatinder is keen to stress that to truly detox, your whole lifestyle has to be adjusted. "Detoxing is not as simple as just eating raw food - it includes being aware of your environment. It means changing your hair gel, your toothpaste, the chemicals you use around the house, chlorinated tap water - even your negative thought patterns. They all introduce toxins into our bodies."

After 12 months of raw food, Jatinder's arthritis all but disappeared. She smiles modestly: "I can now walk and ride a bike for miles, prepare amazing meals and look after my family. And I am pain-free."

From: http://tastymango.com

ANGELA STOKES: ACHIEVED SIGNIFICANT, SUSTAINED AND ENJOYABLE WEIGHT-LOSS – AND CREATED A SUCCESSFUL CAREER IN HEALTH CREATION.

"Half the size, twice the life"

Back in 2002, I was 23 years old, about 19 stone (266lbs/120kg), UK dress size 26-28 and lost in miserable cycles of a non-existent love-life, uncontrollable overeating and complete denial. My pride stopped me discussing my weight with even my closest friends and if anyone tried to broach the subject with me, I strongly resented them for 'interfering'.

My weight had steadily increased since my thyroid gland went under-active aged 11. By 16, I was 16 stone (224lbs/101kg) and my weight increased with my age, a stone a year, until by age 21, at my university graduation in 2000, I was 21 stone (294lbs/133kg). That was the heaviest I reached, and when my health began to suffer so much that I thought I had diabetes, I knew this couldn't continue.

Two summers later I was introduced to the idea that revolutionised my life. A friend lent me 'The Raw Family' by the Boutenkos - a testimonial book about eating mainly or only raw foods for optimum health.[91] I was utterly absorbed - I'd never been interested in diets, health fads or slimming aids and suddenly it seemed the right answer was in my hands. I began the very next day and the improvements in my health over the next weeks were astonishing. You could almost see the weight burn off me - I'll never forget seeing my collar bone again for the first time in years; my skin and hair quality improved dramatically, my energy soared and I was filled with vitality and a new hunger - for real life.

Within a month of going raw, I had my first boyfriend in over 5 years - I was thrilled and increasingly inspired and dedicated to my new lifestyle. As I became less of myself physically, I became more of myself as a whole person. I began to open up in ways that I hadn't found possible before, allowing truth, honesty and trust to develop. I'd been locked up in that body for so long and now the real me was appearing and generating much interest, especially from men.

It's been many years since I started eating raw and I'm happier than I've ever been - I'm now UK dress size 10, can wear whatever clothes I like, eat delicious raw food daily and take great pleasure in treating myself well.

I will always bear the scars of my experiences - physically, my skin is marked, and emotionally and spiritually I experienced great depths of loneliness, depression and insecurity that take time to heal. However, the process has been an extraordinary learning experience and I would not wish to change what I've been through to become the woman I am today.

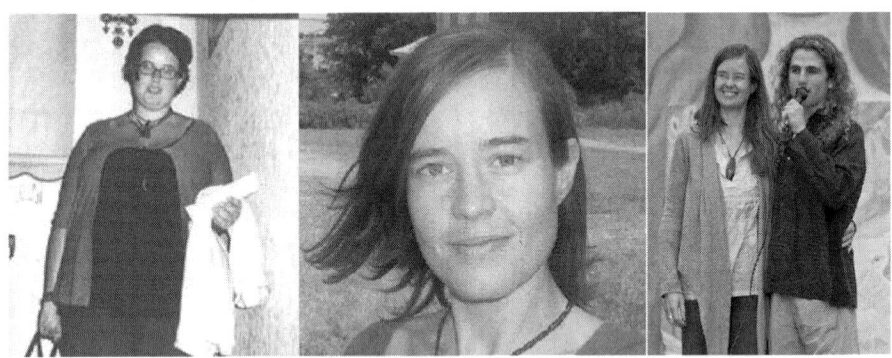

BEFORE - AUG 2001 WEIGHT: 279LBS (APPROX. 20ST/127KG)
AFTER - JULY 2007 WEIGHT: 138LBS (APPROX. 9ST 9LBS/62KG)

From www.rawreform.com – Angela's e-books and seminar tours in the US and UK provide the excellent and inspiring advice on raw foods driven weight-loss. Angela is also now married to another dynamic raw health educator, Matt Monarch, so they form an inspiring team.

---

[91] Victoria Boutenko, *Raw Family*, Raw Family Publishing (2000)

DAVE KLEIN: CURED HIS ULCERATIVE COLITIS

For 25 years David has been enjoying glorious, disease-free health with no medicines or doctoring since completely healing from 8 years of severe ulcerative colitis (1976 - 1984). Since healing up, he has not spent one cent on doctors, medicines or health insurance. Empowering people to gain their health freedom is David's passion and great pleasure in life.

David's Story

My journey into the health education field began in 1975, when at age 17 my robust health began to gradually decline. A heavy eater of meat and junk food, my physical and mental energies deteriorated over a period of six months, then I experienced incessant diarrhoea. After a few weeks of medicine treatment, I showed little improvement, so a colon examination was undertaken. The diagnosis was ulcerative colitis, and I spent my 18th birthday in a hospital, taking prednisone and azulfadine drug treatments. The symptoms subsided, temporarily, but the drugs further ruined my health and had a devastating effect on my mental abilities.

Within a few months, feeling sickly and very weak, I experienced a recurrence of the diarrhea and additional symptoms, including cramping and bleeding, and this lead to further physical deterioration. What ensued were eight tortuous years of colitis flare-ups and off-and-on drug therapy. At age 26, I was reduced to a weak, sickly shadow of my former self. I was having gastric explosions every time I ate, and up to ten painful bowel movements a day with mucus and blood. My nervous system became shattered as I was toxic, debilitated by the medicines, and severely demineralized. Life became a dying hell , but I never gave in to the medical doctors' advice to accept my illness and just be patient until their impossible "miracle drug cure " came along; I desperately wanted my health back and doubted that the doctors were able to help me.

In 1984, I had the great fortune to find a Doctor of Natural Hygiene, Laurence Galant, in Staten Island, who introduced me to the concepts of self-healing and eating a natural plant-based diet. At first I thought the idea of eating raw foods while I was having non-stop diarrhoea was crazy. Yet, I studied Natural Hygiene and slowly cleaned up my diet. I was attached to eating chicken and other favorite cooked foods, however, and was still having colitis flare-ups and relying on medicines.

In the fall of 1984 I had a colonoscopy examination which confirmed that I had advanced ulcerations throughout my sick colon. Surmising that I had been chronically sick and was not getting better, the gastroenterologist recommended that I either try his experimental drug which knocks out the immune system, or have my colon surgically removed. Upon hearing this, a heavy decisive thought entered my mind: I have had it with this medical nightmare - I'll be dead soon if I don't find the answer myself! My life was a gradual descent into hell and now I had to climb out now because I sensed it was almost too late.

Then one amazing night while studying T. C. Fry's Life Science/Natural Hygiene course, I beheld a healing vision and it all made sense. I understood that I was eating a harmful diet which was not compatible with my digestive physiology, and that I needed to eat a plant-based diet with plenty of raw fruits and vegetables - that would allow my body to purge itself of the wastes which were poisoning my colon and preventing me from regaining my health, and would also help me overcome illness and create excellent health. I was ecstatic knowing I had set myself free! The next day I threw away the medicines, divorced myself from all medical intervention for good, gave up all meat and dairy for ever and started a 3-day juice cleanse. By the second day I was coming back to life. On the third day I was feeling better and better and my enthusiasm and joy drove my family and friends crazy! My gut was feeling soothed and I was rejuvenating. I set myself free of illness, doctors and medicines for good, and my bowels were working better and better!!

I adopted a diet with plenty of fruit - that harmonized best with my mind/body/spirit. And with that my energies continuously increased as I detoxified and began rebuilding. Within about six weeks I felt that my colon was completely healed up. I was able to enjoy eating and life again, as my bowels were functioning better than ever. I began a new healthful lifestyle.

Over the next few years I diligently worked at rebuilding my depleted body, incorporating daily running and yoga, all the while studying the life sciences and all of the physical, mental, emotional and spiritual factors which determine our health. It took several years of total dedication to build robust health. In 1993, after a year of study and training at the Institute for Educational Therapy in Cotati, California, I became certified as a Nutrition Educator and began providing nutrition and healing consultations. Today, at age 48, I enjoy excellent health and usually feel fantastic - 22 disease-free years!

From: www.colitis-crohns.com

Since 1993 David Klein, Ph.D. has directed the Colitis & Crohn's Health Recovery Center in Sebastopol, in northern California. David holds a Ph.D. in Health and Natural Healing, is a Hygienic Doctor and is also a Professor with the new University of Natural Health. David is also a Certified Nutrition Educator, offering healing and nutrition consulations – he has counseled over 1,000 people from over 2 dozen countries to new health. David also holds a Bachelor of Science degree in engineering and previously worked in environmental/water quality engineering. He was the editor of *Living Nutrition Magazine*, and now produces its healthy offspring; the eZine *Vibrance*.

SHAZZIE: OVERCAME DEPRESSION, LETHARGY, BRAIN-FOG, PERIOD PAINS, BAD SKIN, & ACHES & PAINS ... TO CREATE A POSITIVE & SUCCESSFUL LIFE SHE LOVES

SHAZZIE'S (Short) BIOGRAPHY – from a past version of www.shazzie.com

Born in East Yorkshire, England, 1969, I grew up with lots of animals, and loved them more than most people! My dog Toby lived for 18 years, and was a brother to me.

In 1985, at the age of 16, I became a vegetarian. 2 years later I was a vegan, after fighting the cheese addiction for a year. Though I was the only vegan I knew, I never regretted sticking with this decision. It suited my feelings towards compassionate living, which was well worth the inconvenience.

Veganism didn't make me any more healthy, though who knows how bad things would have turned out had I continued to consume meat and milk? I'd already suffered a lifetime of feeling isolated, tired and unhappy, so by the time I was an adult this had blossomed into depression, lethargy and brain fog. The physical aches and pains were constant, as was the knowledge that I wasn't living the life I was born to live. In my late 20s, various events caused me to change my life: *for good*.

At the age of 29, I gave up grains for varying lengths of time and ate more salads and fruit. I am convinced this is why my "dive in at the deep end and go into 100% raw food overnight" experience felt like a toe-dip in warm water compared to what some people go through. When I went raw, just before I was 31, I was so ready to change everything that fear had been causing me to hold onto.

Becoming a raw foodist was an intrinsic part of my journey towards mental, spiritual and physical freedom. Out went the house, the job, the country (for a while), the man, and the fear. In came exhilaration. For the first time ever, I was loving life. I felt like I'd been rebuilt in every way. No more crippling period pains, no more bad skin, back ache resolving itself, and finally (thankfully!!) no more depression. I'd been seeking this happiness all my life, and it was all because I decided to only allow positive energy into my body.

Shazzie has built an extremely successful, satisfying and inspiring career in the natural health movement, as a leading raw food advocate, author, educator, programme presenter and entrepreneur with a strong following in the UK, the USA and around the world. She has also been a successful graphic designer and web entrepreneur, and the website she founded www.detoxyourworld.com supplies a wide range of food products, books, equipment and workshops. Her personal website www.shazzie.com also has a strong following, with numerous books, DVDs and e-books and no doubt more on the way, covering raw food, cleansing, recipes and the enjoyment of life, including in the role of a mother – and now also as a Mentor in Business Mastery, sharing her own route to healthy success.

PART 9: THE CONCLUSION

THIS IS THE BEGINNING NOT THE END...

A culture of change is emerging and growing, and in due course it will reach a tipping point. This culture of change immerses itself in the activities, information, attitudes and thinking that naturally take us closer and closer to natural health and sustainability. If you are part of that culture, or want to be, the choices you make about diet and lifestyle are vitally important. To get the best results, your dietary choices and the design of your overall lifestyle need good quality information, thought and careful observation. However, at times you'll need to let go of your thoughts and listen to your body and intuition or gut feelings, to sense what feels 'right' for you, and to gain a deeper sense of what nature, health and sustainability really are.

For me this meant looking at information on raw/living foods, the food industry and nutrition, food growing and my lifestyle in general. It has also involved trusting nature and my body's 'innate intelligence' to tell me what feels good. There is no question that it works.

If you choose to explore an eat more raw path, working with nature as you go, there are many organizations that can help you. If you are looking for greater health and sustainability there are many on the same path, and many sources of information, advice and support.

Much wisdom can be shared between the sustainability and natural health movements, and they are already closely aligned in many ways and through many people. More and more events are combining natural health with ecology and ethical living. There is a way to go before they achieve full alignment, and we fully realize that health and sustainability are one, and that real, whole health means health in every dimension of our inner and outer ecology.

If you need more information on permaculture there are a great range of groups that cover all regions of the USA, or in the UK there's Permaculture Association, which has an extensive network of local groups, activities, courses and an Associated Projects network as well as an excellent newsletter, *Permaculture Works*. A huge number of peoples' lives have been changed very positively by discovering permaculture – in Britain and Europe, in Australia where it started, in the USA, and widely in many of the economically poorer countries around the world, which sometimes can be richer in other ways, with great and inspiring projects in Nepal, India, Africa and South America. Permanent Publications produces the quarterly *Permaculture Magazine* - a superb source of information – and an excellent range of books on permaculture, sustainability and simple living. They also run www.green-shopping.co.uk - a great online shop that covers a vast range of relevant and inter-related subjects and products, including natural health. Both the Association and the Magazine have excellent websites of course, with a large selection of useful and inspiring permaculture links. Chelsea Green in the USA produce and sell a similarly excellent range of sustainable living books, and *Permaculture Design Magazine* (formerly *Permaculture Activist*) is a great starting place to find your way into the north American permaculture world.

Similarly there is a wealth of raw food information available - I've referred to a good number of these individuals and organizations throughout this book, and summarise a range of contacts in the Appendices. Thanks to such individuals and organisations, and despite what I thought before 1994, I now know that I can survive and thrive, be healthier and happier on a high raw foods diet – AND, I can grow a lot more of my own food than I would have thought possible years ago, both organically and at very low cost.

Personally, I sense we are at or are approaching what author Malcolm Gladwell has termed a 'tipping point'.[92] This is coming in many areas, as people and social movements wake up to the realities of climate change, and the downward spirals of unsustainability and ill-health. As ecological scientist-philosopher Fritjof Capra says, *'the significant crises we face in the world, 'are all facets of one and the same crisis, and this is a crisis of perception'*. This manifests in the same patterns of thinking in the health and nutrition fields, and the agriculture and food industry fields, as well as in politics, education and the media – all producing a wide range of inter-related problems. Capra emphasizes that the Chinese symbol for *crisis* is composed of the symbols for *danger* and *opportunity* – so crisis always contains opportunity. Thus, more people are aware that *upward spirals towards health and sustainability are available now*, and that our fate lies in our own hands. If we change how we perceive and think about health and food, we can change our actions and effects in the world, and problems can be turned to solutions. In every significant area our life those solutions are facets of the same solution - which is a fundamental change in our understanding of ourselves and the world that we are a part of - a change of sufficient depth that it leads to different thinking, different actions and different results in all areas.

As Einstein said, *'the significant problems of our time cannot be solved at the same level of thinking that created them – we have to move to a new level of thinking'*. This requires us to evolve and up-grade many behaviours, beliefs, modes of understanding and patterns of thinking to transform our activities to achieve much improved outcomes. At the same time, the use of forms of positive communication is growing (e.g. non-violent communication). The movement to natural child birth and natural parenting is becoming stronger (see *The Mother* magazine), and more and more people are recognizing these interconnected strands of the sane, humane and ecological path.[93] If you follow this path, and choose the upward spiral, you'll find the same set of ecological ethics and principles can be used to guide your diet and lifestyle as a whole.

Either consciously or unconsciously, you do a lot of designing of your lifestyle – work and career, image and pastimes, home and garden, mode of transport, and of course the food you eat. In designing your own lifestyle you can base your food and health choices on good quality information, on careful observation and actual experience. In this way, by working with nature you can design a lifestyle that is more positive, more sustainable and more naturally healthy.

This may mean challenging your preconceptions and delving deep into changes in your lifestyle. At the same time, you can cut down on TV and newspapers, replacing them with positive, healthy and creative nutrition for your mind, spirit and emotions – helpful and enjoyable books, magazines, DVD's, CDs and tapes, websites, on-line videos and downloads, networks and friends. 'What the Bleep', 'Supersize Me', 'The Secret', 'Age of Stupid', 'Dirt!', 'Time of the Sixth Sun', '11th Hour' ... these are all evidence of a wider social turning point. We are at least becoming more aware of the depth of the problem. The next step will be more and more films focused on

---

[92] Malcolm Gladwell, *The Tipping Point: how little things can make a big difference*, Little Brown, 2000: an excellent and important book.

[93] See http://www.themothermagazine.co.uk/

turning the problems to solutions. And as this shift occurs, what we can broadly call the *eat more raw lifestyle* and *real health creation* is being seen as having an important role in lubricating that turning point, creating a change of culture and a culture of change.

SHIFT FROM CONSUMING LIFE TO PRODUCING HEALTH

If we link agroforestry, local organic growing, forest gardening, the Plants For A Future concept, permaculture thinking, indoor gardening, intuitive eating and an understanding of raw food nutrition, with a dose of Food For Free, it can provide us with the tools to take the first steps towards creating a new, liberated, vibrant and vital, health-creating, sustainable and life-enhancing culture. You can use these tools on your path as you move to your own tipping point.

You can change what you buy and how you use money. You can buy food and products that support moves towards greater health, in yourself and in the ecological health of the planet. You can spend and invest only in ways which create greater health and sustainability. You can buy foods with minimum packaging, and cut out tinned foods and other over packaged foods. You can buy from farm shops, or organic veggie box schemes. You can buy dried seeds and pulses, and dried fruit, and again reduce the packaging in your waste stream. And you can seek friends and like-minded people, learning together how to do it from others who have done so elsewhere. And at the same time you can grow more of your own food.

You can also ensure that your work is making a positive contribution to resolving or transforming the significant problems of our time, rather than adding to them. There's an awful lot of positive work that still needs to be done in health creation, sustainability and numerous fields. Our work is normally our greatest contribution to the economy, so if you are being a conscious consumer but an unconscious worker ... well, that's missing the point. Move beyond the reasons and justifications not to change, and move into the reality that numerous people have already made the shift, and in many cases become more successful or much more fulfilled as a result – and sometimes both. It's our work that is creating the future that we are living into, much more so than what we consume - so work to create a positive future, rather than working to sustain a present that is not solving the problems, but just adding to them.

Get planting! Buy some seeds, plants and trees for your garden, allotment, or for a community garden. 'Plant, Plant, Plant' in your own patch an all year vegetable, herb and salad garden; plant a forest garden – anything from a tiny mini-forest garden to a huge edible forest will do. Every little does help. Every action has its effect, either one way or another ... or another! Choose positive, creative effects and love every minute of it!

Plant liberally and carefully in your landscape. Plant many types of plants and seeds. Liberally plant and sow ideas, information, actions and visions of a more healthy and sustainable future. Sow seeds in your own life, by making changes yourself. *Be part of the culture of change*, bringing more and more tipping points towards health, sustainability and a wiser world into your life and our culture as a whole. Co-create, diversify and expand the growing, living library of natural diversity of ideas, actions and visions. 'Plant, Plant, Plant' in your lifestyle and along your path to create real health, to transform your patch, your local area and the whole living landscape to create productive, healthy and sustainable living systems.

It may not be easy, but it's got to be worth a try. Now it's over to you...

PART 10: RECIPES, FOOD PREPARATION AND MEAL IDEAS

There are many raw food recipe books containing a host of wonderful dishes, both savoury and sweet, to entice the palate, to boggle the eyes and to make the taste buds dance with joy. To get you off to a good start, in this section you have a full range of basic recipes which are easy to prepare and usually scrumptiously delicious, as well as providing fantastic nutrition. Is that your mouth watering already?!

Although there's a great selection of recipes this section isn't trying to compete with the various glossy recipe books that are out there. It's aiming to be more practical than that, and to give you more of a handbook for getting going and learning some 'tricks of the trade'. Because most of us use recipe books as the exception, not the rule. For breakfast, lunch and supper 7 days a week, mostly we need the basics, not the glossy cordon bleu stuff – so that's my focus here, the practical day-to-day stuff. Once you've got the basics, raw food preparation is generally simpler than cooking, usually with less preparation time and certainly with less and easier clearing up than cooked meals. You don't need a whole bunch of complicated raw recipes – although if you want them there are plenty of them out there, with 'Cordon Raw' now very fashionable in California, London and New York, for example.

Just as in conventional eating, most people rely on a few basic recipes which they rotate and vary. So with this good set of standard meals you're more than half way there. And once you've started more options and choices will come your way.

The aim here is to get you started, although, most of all I want you to feel confident about experimenting and creating your own favourite meals – which is actually easy once you've got the hang of it. Personally I tend not to use exact quantities but follow my own instinct on how much of what to include. This way I get different proportions of ingredients, which means it tastes deliciously different every time. So some of the donated recipes below include measurements, and others do not. Later, in the Appendices section, there's a list of on-line stores to help you source more extensive recipe books, foods, equipment and courses.

STEVE'S RECIPE FOR SUCCESS

Keep a good selection of fruit and salad vegetables through the week (home grown and/or bought), then choose each day according to what you fancy. Use 5 to 15 basic salad ingredients, then play around with different proportions and mixtures, using the additional flavours suggested below for variety as you like. Some days you can leave out one, two or three ingredients, and on other you can leave out a whole bunch and just have a really simple mix of your favourites. Other days you can add a whole bunch more.

So here's a list of different salad ingredients you can go for:
- Salad leaves and cabbage family: kale and cabbage (red, white, green); rocket; lettuce (particularly Romaine); spinach; oriental greens (mitzuna, etc); chicory/endive; wild greens and perennial greens – mixed salad packs if you are buying.
- Roots: carrots; beetroot/beets; kohl rabi; parsnip; onions; sweet potato; turnip.

- Veg Fruit: tomatoes; cucumbers; courgette/zucchini; red or yellow sweet/bell pepper.[94]
- Other Veg: celery; broccoli; cauliflower, etc.
- Avocados.
- Sprouts: alfalfa, green lentils, radish, mixed sprouts, etc.

Flavourings: On the side, the following can be useful to help the transition to an eat more raw lifestyle: sea weed (e.g. dulse), olive oil, garlic, spices (cayenne/chilli, cumin, etc.), ginger.

Often, the simpler the better – try not to get 'addicted' to strong stimulating flavours, enjoy them, yes, and at the same time make sure you have regular simple meals without them. Adding lemon juice brings out flavours and helps prevent oxidation of foods. Cold pressed olive oil and salty flavours (e.g. tamari) are also often helpful in making a transition from a normal diet to one which is 'high raw'. Apple cider vinegar is a great alternative to lemon juice, particularly for temperate or cooler climates. Balsamic is another option.

Equipment: add to your basic ingredients a good knife and chopping board, a grater and perhaps one or two gadgets like a hand mincer and hand seed grinder, a good and ideally beautiful bowl or plate or two that you enjoy eating from, and then you're away...! You can definitely get by with basic blenders and juicers (I did for years), if you're on a low income (as I was for many of my raw years). Although if you can afford it good equipment will do a better job.

SOME REALLY DELICIOUS AND RADICALLY HEALTHY RECIPES

Many of these recipes have been donated by friends and contacts who support the 'eat more raw' philosophy and way of life, and who have all traveled the road of transition – so thanks to you all. They know how to prepare meals that taste great, whilst also helping our minds and bodies get used to eating differently. Where relevant, and as a rough but helpful guide, the recipes are marked as 'Eco' if they are likely to be particularly suited to unprocessed, local and / or easily grown foods, in temperate or Mediterranean-type climates, and depending on the seasonality of foods.

For most working people and school kids / students what we need is breakfast and lunch options that are simple, quick and easy. For most people the evening meal is the main meal during the week (main meal recipes follow shortly), whilst the following suggestions for breakfast and lunch are really practical, simple and quick ways to get yourself off to a really good start, and keep that going through the main part of the day.

Some recipes are described as '**Eco**', which simply indicates that when eaten in the climate where the ingredients are produced they will be both healthy should be ecologically sound, hopefully available locally grown and with low food miles. '**Eco Med**' indicates it being ecologically good for a Mediterranean / sub-tropical climate.

---

[94] I suggest you do not use green peppers as they are unripe red or yellow peppers – remember, ripe simply means 'ready to eat', whilst unripe means 'not ready to eat'.

BREAKFAST AND MORNING

Vary between any of the following, or stick with your favourites:
- Fruit only breakfast / Fruit snacks through the morning - or a dried fruit and seeds / nuts snack for late morning – seasonal and climatically appropriate local/regional fruit make this a very eco option;
- Freshly made juice - especially with celery, greens, etc (e.g. carrot, apple and celery is a great basic juice) **(eco)**;
- Raw muesli;
- Freshly made hemp / seed / nut milk (can include nettles / greens, or super foods to 'up' the power of this fantastic food even further) – put all the ingredients in a blender with spring water, blend well and then strain **(eco)**;
- Super-nutrient breakfast pudding: 1 cup + soaked figs / raisins / dates, blended with 1 cup + soaked pumpkin, flax and sunflower seeds / walnuts, plus all or any of the following: approx. 20 drops of Marine Minerals' liquid ionic trace minerals, 1-2 tsp of maca powder, 1-2 tsp barley greens / green superfoods powder, high quality vitamin B12 supplement, tbsp flax / hemp oil, 1 tbsp raw cacao, 2 tsp carob powder, etc, and a little spring water if needed – this is fantastic for children and for pregnant / nursing mothers – serves 2+ depending on appetites / size etc – you can also add orange peel, orange / apple / banana, and a *small* quantity of herb salt if needed - note: you can make twice as much as you need and keep it in the fridge for a day;
- 'Dada Porridge' as it's known in my house: banana, a little lemon or orange juice, pumpkin seed, flax seed, sunflower seed, raisins, goji berries, flax oil and water – varients include adding raw cacao nibs, blueberries, apple or pear, date, fig or whatever else takes my fancy;
- Smoothie – a variation on the breakfast pudding recipes above, with more fresh fruit and with or without smaller quantities of soaked seeds / nuts or dried fruit;

Note 1: the nutrient-dense pudding recipes are excellent for brain building for young and older alike, particularly the super-nutrient breakfast pudding.

Note 2: having a heavy breakfast of unsoaked nuts / dried fruit etc will create too much work for the body in the early part of the day, so it's good to keep breakfast lighter and if nuts and seeds are used they should be soaked or blended with fruit and / or water. I tend to move towards the puddings in autumn and winter, but usually find them too heavy at other times of the year.

Ideally drink water when you get up, before you have breakfast – and if you're using green superfoods drinks, also have these before any breakfast meal.

Morning Glory (Eco Med) – from Dave Klein, Living Nutrition Magazine
- Several sweet oranges.
- 1 pomegranate.

Slice the oranges and pomegranate in half, use citrus juicer, then mix and enjoy!

Grape – Celery Cooler (Eco Med) – from Dave Klein, Living Nutrition Magazine

Juice your favourite sweet grapes. After the grapes, juice 1 or 2 celery stalks per glass. Stir and serve. Garnish with mint leaves if desired. Optional: Cut a thin slice of fresh ginger root. Juice the ginger slice with the grapes.

Practical Working Lunch / School Lunch

A selection from the following will see you through the day, and make a great difference to your afternoon energy levels:

- Mix of dried fruit and nuts / seeds e.g. brazils, almonds, cashews, raisins, figs, pumpkin, sunflower;
- 1, 2 or several fruits, ideally seasonal and local **(eco)**;
- Salad mixed with soaked seeds (use a re-usable container of a size that suits your needs) include for example variations of the following: romaine lettuce, rocket, sliced red onion, grated carrot / beetroot / kohlrabi, dressing (ideally lemon juice and flax oil), sliced cucumber/celery etc **(eco)**;
- Chunk of cucumber / stick of celery / sticks of carrot **(eco)**;
- Raw snack bar e.g. Yaoh, Gillian McKeith, Supergreens, etc;
- Dehydrated crackers (e.g. flax crackers).

OTHER SIMPLE SNACK LUNCH OPTIONS

Avo-buttered Corn On The Cob (Eco Med) – from Dave Klein, Living Nutrition Magazine
- Fresh Corn on the cob.
- Avocado.

Smear the avocado over the corn and enjoy! Best eaten barefoot!

Sesame Hors d'Oeuvres – from Dave Klein, Living Nutrition Magazine **(Eco Med)**
- Raw sesame tahini.
- Slicing cucumbers.

Slice the cucumbers into discs or length-ways (if the skins are waxed, peeling is mandatory). Spoon tahini on the cuke slices. Optional: place another cucumber slice on top of the tahini, to make a mini sandwich.

SAVOURY DISHES FROM AROUND THE WORLD

THREE ORIENTAL DISHES
Oriental Meal: Spring Rolls & Satay Sauce

Spring Rolls - you can grow your own bean sprouts, or buy them. Homegrown are more nutritious, although for some people, shop bought sprouts will make the whole thing look better!
- 1 or 2 cloves of garlic – finely chopped or put through garlic press
- A piece of fresh ginger – grated or finely chopped
- ½ a red onion or sliced spring onion
- small bunch coriander / cilantro, and / or parsley, chives etc.
- 1 carrot and / or parsnip or celeriac
- ½ a red or yellow sweet / bell pepper
- 1 or 2 handfulls of bean sprouts
- tamari
- apple cider vinegar
- Olive oil
- Large leaves of Spring cabbage, white/red cabbage or Romaine (Cos) lettuce

Mix together the garlic, ginger and onion. Grate the carrot / root veg, slice the sweet pepper and chop the coriander / greens. Transfer everything (apart from the large leaves) to a bowl, and mix. Then spoon the filling on to your leaves, and roll them up carefully, as the mix can easily spill out – practice makes perfect, as they say!

Satay Sauce - a very popular sauce, with many variations amongst raw chefs. You can try this in all sorts of dishes, so the suggestion of a noodle version is just one amongst many options.
- 2 or 3 dates
- 1/2 cup raw tahini or almond butter
- 1/4 cup raw coconut butter
- 1 tablespoon tamari
- 1 teaspoon fresh grated ginger
- 1 tablespoon olive oil
- Juice from 1 lemon
- 2 cloves garlic, chopped / through garlic press
- 1 teaspoon chili powder / flakes or chopped raw chilli
- Soaked sundried tomato
- Sweet / bell pepper (red or yellow)
- Pinch of herb salt / Himalayan Salt

Noodles
- Courgettes / zucchini and / or large carrots, 'spiralized' into noodles
- 1 cup mange tout / chopped snow pea pods
- Spring onions / chopped red onion / scallions, sliced

Blend together dates, coconut butter, tahini / almond butter, tamari, ginger, olive oil, and lemon juice until smooth. Then add garlic, chili and Himalayan, and briefly mix / pulse to blend. Pour over carrot noodle mixture, mix well and enjoy!

Sushi (thanks to Matri & Lucho at Cana Dulce – www.permaculturacanadulce.org) Soak pumpkin seeds overnight, then blend into a thick mix with with stoned olives, a little lemon juice, olive oil, and tamari, as well coriander / cilantro, some red pepper and ground black pepper. Paste the mix on Nori sheets and then add a thin layer of grated carrot, finely chopped red onion and celery. Roll it all up, leaving an uncovered edge of Nori to seal the roll with a little water. Slice into pieces and serve. Grate any white vegetable for a rice effect.

Noodle dishes can be easily created with the help of a 'spiraliser' used on courgettes, parsnip, daikon or other white vegetables. Mung **bean sprouts**, and many other sprouts, can be used in a wide range of dishes. **Sweet and sour sauces** can be created by blending soaked dates, lemon juice, apple cider vinegar, sweet pepper and sundried tomatoes, with a variety of other ingredients added to vary the sweet and sour flavour. Try the dishes with walnuts or pecans for a slightly heavier variation.

THREE MIDDLE EASTERN DISHES
Raw Chickpea Humous
Organic dried chickpeas, soaked overnight and then sprouted for between 1 and 3 days. Use a hand mincer / blender / food processor to combine chickpeas and garlic, and some water if using the blender. Then mix in lemon juice and olive oil. Depending on what I have available, and who I'm preparing it for (i.e. those who are on a 'normal' diet tend to want a bit more of the salty flavours).

Other tastes you can add to the humous:
- Salty element (desirable for many, but not essential): celery or chard stalks, seaweed, dried tomatoes, miso, tamari – or if you are still using salt then good quality seasalt.
- Seeds: linseed/flax, ground sesame (not soaked before hand), sunflower, hemp, pumpkin (ideally soaked before hand) – or if you prefer you can add tahini (ideally raw, but which normally is difficult to obtain raw).
- Chopped herbs to mix in or sprinkle on top when blended or minced.
- Chilli (preferably fresh raw or sundried), ginger or other hot ingredients to spice it up when I feel like it.
- Finely chopped tomato and/or onion can be added on some days.
- Sometimes, if I'm a bit low on chickpeas and it needs filling out, or if I fancy a flavour change, I might add some carrot, squash/pumpkin or parsnip.
- And dried *Ginkgo biloba* leaves (harvested from the local park and dried oneself ideally!) – a very beneficial herb for the brain and circulation, not an essential ingredient by any means, but this is the permaculture of nutrition, so why not regularly add some into your humous or salad to get maximum benefit with minimum effort!

Humous is a delicious and cheap base for salads in cooler climates, where avocados (which are another favourite base for salad dishes) might be out of the price range and ecologically less desirable (due to their 'food miles') – and it's also great for warmer climates. It is great with dips, with salads or in 'real salad sandwiches' – humous and other ingredients rolled up or folded in a spring cabbage, Romaine lettuce or kale leaf.

Falafel Patties
This is slightly adapted from Frederic Paténaude's excellent book *Sunfood Cuisine*[95]. It is a favourite dish that is expertly produced by Joe and Carme, great raw friends previously in southern Spain and now in Brazil.
- 1.1/2 cups of sprouted lentils or chick peas.
- 1 cup sprouted sunflower seeds.
- 1 tablespoon minced garlic.
- 2 cups fresh cilantro/coriander, chopped (or a tablespoon in powder form).
- 1/2 cup fresh parsley.
- 1/2 cup sesame seeds (or raw tahini).
- Salty element according to taste, not too much though (seaweed, minced or chopped chard stalks or celery).
- 1/2 cup chopped onion.
- 1/2 cup freshly squeezed lemon juice.
- 1/4 cup olive oil.
- 1.1/2 teaspoons ground cumin seed, or powder.

Combine all ingredients using a hand mincer or blender, and then have fun forming a blended mixture into small patties. Leave them in a sunny or warm place (ideally in direct sunlight) to dry or dehydrate for up to 8 hours.

Marinated Aubergines (thanks to Matri and Lucho at Cana Dulce – www.permaculturacanadulce.org)
Peel 3 aubergines (egg plant) and slice thinly length-ways, then sprinkle with a little salt to remove any bitterness. Mix olive oil, crushed garlic, parsley, tamari and lemon juice and then marinate the aubergine slices for 8 hours / overnight in this mix. To make the dish, use two layers with a tomato or mixed veg sauce with sprouted lentils at the base and in between, and a white sauce layer on top (made from blending together soaked sunflower seeds, a small amount of linseed, olive oil or flax/omega oil, a little lemon juice and garlic, with a little seasoning) spinkled with a ground linseed / dried brewer's yeast mix. It's very filling!

---

[95] Frederic Patenaude, *Sunfood Cuisine*, Nature's First Law (2002)

Three Curry Dishes

Chris' Raw Curry (thanks to Chris Kennett at Veggie Power - www.veggiepower.co.uk)
This can be a real eye-opener and taste-teaser for normal eaters and raw foodies alike. A genuine tasting, delicious raw curry... wow!

- Many ingredients: avocado, red or other onions (according to your taste preferences), chopped / grated carrots, some chopped cauliflower stem, some soaked dates (make a real difference), lemon juice, and any other chopped veg you feel like throwing in.
- Fresh coconut, or organic coconut butter / creamed coconut is a great addition;
- Spices and flavour: cumin seeds (the key to the genuine curry flavour), curry powder, ginger, garlic, chilli/cayenne, etc.
- **Raw 'Rice'** base**: cauliflower, chopped very fine or put through food processor or a hand mincer. Other white ingredients can also be used either with or instead of cauliflower, such as white cabbage or radish/mouli, as well as additional flavoring ingredients such as ginger, coriander/cilantro leaf, cumin seed.

Mix or hand mince the main curry ingredients, spices and flavours together, ideally by hand-mincer or using a food processor rather than a blender, so that you have lots of chunky bits. Finely chop the cauliflower using a hand-mincer or food processor, or finely chop by hand, to create the fine white 'rice' bed and then serve the curry on top or at the side, with other side dishes (e.g. cucumber) and garnished as you wish. It looks great and it's delicious!

Amanda's Sweet (not hot) Curry Sauce - can be used with raw rice** above
Blend or hand mince together tomatoes, carrots or pumpkin/squash, olive oil, desiccated coconut or some creamed coconut block (not a whole block!), mild curry powder and other curry spices and / or a little garlic if you wish.

Funky Raw Curry Sauce - can be used with raw rice** above (thanks to Rob, www.funkyraw.com)

- 2 sundried tomatoes (soaked)
- 4 tomatoes
- 1 carrot
- handful fresh coriander
- 1 wild garlic leaf (you can of course use shop bought garlic if you prefer!)
- 1/2 tsp dried coriander
- 1/2 tsp cumin
- 1/4 tsp fenugreek
- 1/2 tsp tumeric
- 1/2 tsp garam masala

Put all ingredients into your blender, including a little soak water from the dried tomatoes and blend.

Three Mexican and South American Dishes

Guacamole (Eco Med) - Very popular and simple – avocados mashed or blended with a range of other ingredients: garlic and lemon juice are the two basic essentials, although finely chopped tomato and onion/chives are also often added. I find that adding different herbs like dill, parsley and coriander/cilantro on different occasions adds to the fun of experimenting with dishes that are always delicious anyway! A bit of chilli and/or ginger gives it some extra zing if you like it like that. Have it with a big salad of mixed leaves.

Raw Tacos (Eco Med) (thanks to Matri and Lucho at Cana Dulce – www.permaculturacanadulce.org) - Chop up and mix together: Red pepper, red/spring onion or leek (a very strong flavour when raw, so use sparingly), shredded lettuce or other greens, diced tomato, coriander and / or parsley, avocado – a little olive oil and chilli are optional. You can make a sauce from blended seeds, fresh / sundried tomatoes, garlic, lemon juice, olive oil, etc. Scoop into a large cabbage or romaine lettuce leaf – or possible a large kale or chard leaf - fold over or roll up and enjoy.

January's Sprouted Quinoa Salads - this January is a lively long term UK raw food chef and teacher who does some amazing things with sprouted Quinoa! Quinoa is one of those fantastic foods that most people think you have to cook; but you don't. Soak it for a few hours, or overnight, then drain it off and you'll almost be able to watch those little sprouts grow before your eyes. Rinse and drain them once a day, and they are ready from 2 to 3 days, but don't last well beyond that. They are very healthy sprouts. January's Quinoa salads vary enormously and are always delicious: tomato, a little red onion, some seaweed, celery, a little lemon juice, some fresh herbs... whatever takes your fancy. The great thing about sprouting Quinoa (organic of course) is that it is so simple, quick and cheap, and a totally reliable basis for a sprouted salad.

Two Italian Dishes

Raw Lasagna (Seasonally Eco)
Slice courgette/zucchini into long strips to form 'pasta' slices. Make a blended sauce of tomatoes, olive oil and basil, with chopped red onion and a little mixed herbs added in – soaked dried tomatoes will make the sauce much richer; added herb salt / sea salt to taste.
Blend together soaked sunflower, pumpkin and flax seed, with garlic and a little oil to create a fine 'white' sauce. Mix soaked walnuts or sprouted lentils into the tomato sauce (chopped olives are another optional extra) and then layer this followed by white sauce and then 'pasta' two or three sets of layers deep. Ground linseed (or a little dried brewer's yeast) can be sprinkled on the top.

Raw Spaghetti and other Raw Pastas (Seasonally Eco)
It's possible to find specialized food slicers, graters, etc which enable you to make thin strings from courgette, squash and other vegetables (one is the rather expensive but fun Saladeco 'Spiralizer'). With this you can make raw spaghetti creating a variation on the lasagna recipe above. You can experiment with grating, slicing and chopping these vegetables in different ways to make various pasta dishes. Basil and pine nuts can be blended together to make a raw pesto.

OTHER DISHES

Stuffed Tomatoes, Peppers, Mushrooms or Avocados (Seasonally Eco)

You can vary the contents and the container. Fillings can include grated root vegetables or squash, shredded lettuce / leaves, diced avocado, herbs, mixes with soaked seeds or nuts, grated cauliflower, sprouted lentils or chickpeas, and a range of seasonings. Fill the container with the veg mix and serve with a tomato sauce - or one of the other sauce recipes.

Seed / Nut Patés

There are variations on the basic seed paté recipe, and my experience is that they are often very popular with non-rawfooders. Soaked seeds are best, which usually will be organic hemp, sunflower or pumpkin, all or any of them – soaked nuts can also be used. These should be put through the hand grinder or mincer, the blender or a masticating juicer with the non-juicing attachment. Ground dry linseed/flax seeds are a good addition which will thicken up the blend, and of course sesame can be used too. If you haven't soaked your main seed ingredients then dry seeds can be put through a grinder (hand or electric). To these can be added other ingredients, with the two keys being lemon juice to bring up the flavour and prevent oxidation, and a salty element, which may be any of those mentioned in the Humous recipe above.

These additional ingredients can include fresh or dried herbs, tomatoes, mushrooms and all sorts of other ingredients – I find that red / yellow peppers, red/Spanish onions and dried tomato are particularly excellent paté ingredients. Include chilli or ginger to spice it up if you like that. You should not use more than 100 grammes (3-4 ounces) or so of seeds per person, so it works well to add in the minced vegetables with the seeds to bulk it up. Add more watery ingredients carefully so that the paté does not get sloppy.* Put everything together through a hand mincer or food processor. If you experiment you'll find your own favourite paté mixes.

With this paté recipe (and the dip recipes that follow) you can use carrot/cucumber/celery/courgette(zucchini) sticks, lettuce/chicory leaves, cauliflower, broccoli, dehydrated crackers ... all sorts of things.

* Note: Ground Linseed is a great ingredient to use to thicken up savoury or sweet dishes alike, if they get a bit sloppy.

Seed / Nut Dips

Follow the same process as for paté but use more liquid ingredients, particularly tomatoes, and / or add some spring water to get a less solid consistency, that works well as a dip.

Raw Coleslaw

This is another dish that goes down well at parties and gatherings, and I've had many non-rawfooders tell me that my coleslaw is the best they ever had! Thinly slice white and / or red cabbage and red onion, add grated carrot and mix. Make a white dressing with sunflower, pumpkin and flax seed blended with water, apple cider vinegar, oil, lemon juice and garlic – adding some sundried tomato and / or red pepper to the blended sauce also works very well. Mix together and ideally leave to stand for a few hours before eating, though this is far from essential. Add chopped chives, coriander / cilantro and / or other herbs.

Real 'Salad Sandwiches' (Eco)
Similar to the raw tacos ... Take any range of salad ingredients and savoury dishes and heap them into a large cabbage leaf, romaine lettuce leaf, kale leaf, chard leaf or whatever else may be available. Fold over or roll up and enjoy.

Basic Green Salad
Romaine or other lettuce leaves; sliced red onion; spinach, coriander / cilantro, etc if available; chopped or sliced avocado; alfalfa sprouts; other sald leaves fresh from the garden (rocket, saladini, etc); squeeze of lemon juice and simple dressing – mix it about a little then serve with other dishes. Yum.

Raw Mayonnaise - (thanks Matri & Lucho, Cana Dulce – wwwpermaculturacanadulce.org) blend together soaked sunflower seeds, with a little linseed, with water, garlic, olive oil and herb/sea salt.

Caramelised Onions (thanks Matri & Lucho, Cana Dulce – permaculturacanadulce.org)
Ingredients: Onions, dates (soaked), tamari.
Slice onions very finely and leave to soak in a little water for ½ hour, then remove and rinse, keeping the soak water. Blend the dates with some soak water (from dates and onions) and the tamari. Marinate the onions in the sauce for at least 6 hours.
Serving suggestions: with raw burgers (see below), in raw tacos or sandwiches, on top of stuffed tomatoes, peppers, avocados or mushrooms. Or simply as a side dip with a large salad.

RAW SOUPS

Watercress and Garlic Soup (from Holly Paige, www.rawcuisine.co.uk and Funky Raw magazine)
- 1 big handful watercress
- 2 tomatoes
- 1 avocado
- 1 tablespoon or 15 ml lemon juice

1 or 2 cloves garlic
1 sun-dried tomato
2 teaspoons or 10ml flax oil
1 ½ pints water

Blend all ingredients until smooth. A high-speed blender gives particularly creamy soup.

Gaspacho
Blend together lots of tomatoes with celery, garlic and coriander, as well as olive (or flax) oil or a bit of avocado for a thicker soup. Finely chopped red onion can also be added.

Other Raw Soups
Raw soups can be made from a variety of ingredients, and green soups are particularly nutritious e.g. with spinach, kale, broccoli, romaine lettuce, watercress, etc. Vegetables with a high liquid content (e.g. tomatoes, cucumber, celery, red pepper) are also excellent, although spring water can also be used. Grated carrot, beetroot etc can also be an option. Add a salty element and an oily/fatty element (e.g. olive/flax/hemp oil, soaked seeds, avocado) for a satisfying soup, with other flavourings (e.g. pepper, chilli, cumin) added as required. Use 5 to 10 main ingredients max.

Sundried (in a warm climate) or Dehydrator Dishes

A dehydrator is very much an option, and not an essential. It can be helpful for getting to 50:50 raw, or in transition to a high raw diet.

Flax Crackers - Proportions: 1 cup soaked flax seeds (can also add a little of other seeds), blended with carrot and / or celery, mixed with 1 cup ground dry flax seeds and finely chopped red onion / chives. Add herb salt, pepper, etc. to the mix according to taste, and dehydrate overnight. You can make much larger quantities to keep in an air tight container for several days / 1 week.

Raw Vegi-Burgers (thanks Matri & Lu at Cana Dulce – www.permaculturacanadulce.org) **(Eco)** - Mix together lentil sprouts, chopped onion, olive oil, stoned olives, parsley / herbs, grated carrot/squash and tamari. Mix in enough ground linseed to make the mixture firm enough to make into flattened 'burgers'. Place in the sun for up to four hours, or dehydrate overnight.

Seed Bread / Crackers
- Grated carrots, beetroot, etc
- Finely chopped red onion
- 4 seeds – 3 cup linseed soaked, 2 cup hemp soaked, 3-4 cup dry mix of Linseed, sunflower, pumpkin, sesame.

Blend together less than ½ of the seed mix with a little water then mix with all the other ingredients, potentially also including herbs and other ingredients to taste (garlic, chilli, etc). Add sundried tomatoes and sweet pepper to the blended ingredients for a great flavor. Dehydrate overnight to make a large quantity that can be kept in an air tight container.

A Culinary Tip – two versions of 'The 5 Tastes'

This secret of success is evidently part'n'parcel of the conventional culinary arts, as well as raw foods cuisine.
- Victoria Bountenko's recipe success is based significantly on combining five key flavours, in very varying mixes, from savoury dishes to sweets. Those five flavours are: Sweet, Sour, Salty, Spicey and Bitter;
- A variation on this (promoted by Holly Paige in the Funky Raw network) is to combine the following: Fat, Salty, Acid, Pungent (e.g. cumin), Sweet.

The point is that if all these tastes are included as elements of a dish then all the tastes are stimulated and satisfied by the meal.

Other Savoury Dishes for Anywhere and Everywhere

Turner's Field T'rific Green Salad (Eco) - the idea of this recipe is that once you've read this book you'll go out and grow a whole lot of these plants in your garden, allotment, window box, a friend or any place you can get your hands on. This salad involves walking round the garden, preferably barefoot, picking all or any of the following that can be combined into a green salad of unbelievable vibrancy and deliciousness! It's also great to take children round to help

you, giving them the chance to taste (with care, as some tastes are strong) and see each of the plants as you go:
- Rocket, perpetual spinach, perennial onion leaves, perennial or annual broccoli (leaves and/or sprouts), perennial or annual kale, chives, lemon balm, sorrel, landcress, lovely lovage, parsley, *Peltaria*/garlic cress, campanula, sweet cicely, fennel, thyme, garlic chives, leek leaves, dandelions, with some finely chopped sage or rosemary, and if its spring or early summer ransoms and hedge garlic (Jack-by-the-Hedge), oriental salad leaves and so on. That's what I call a salad!

And if you want a lettuce then Romaine is great, or try Black Seeded Simpson's for something more unusual. The final vital and vibrant ingredient that gives it that special touch is a few (or loads!) of whatever flowers are available: borage, calendula, chives, mallow, lavateria, nasturtiums, and so on (most of you will probably want to remember to shake the little bugs out of the flowers as you go!). There is nothing quite like a flower-festooned salad to bring beauty to the meal.

Ariadne's Wolf-Up (Eco) - this is a serious power-pack of a dish, and is a favourite of Ariadne Fern (of the project Plants for a Future), who is a trained nutritionist. It really gives me a tremendous feeling of vitality and strength. But it's not for the faint hearted because whilst many people love it, others find it too powerful. It is designed to be packed with chlorophyll as well as including seeds that contain particular 'essential' amino acids. Wolf-up involves picking a lot of wild greens and salad greens (e.g. kale) and then putting these through a hand mincer (some of which look like a wolf's head in profile, hence the name) or a masticating juicer with the non-juicing attachment. Add to the greens ground hemp, sunflower, pumpkin and/or flax seeds, and some lemon juice and garlic if required. Some celery or chard stems will add a 'salty' element to the flavour. If you find it too powerful to start with try less wild greens – it's worth experimenting as it's a dish that can really grow on you.

SOME OTHER STAPLES AND GREAT SALAD DISHES

- Grated carrot with orange and ginger makes a great combination of flavours.
- Raw grated beetroot/beets is fantastic as it is, or with just a dash of olive oil, lemon juice or apple cider vinegar - beetroot/beet is easy to grow in a good rich soil.
- Grated parsnip with chopped leek, green onions or plenty of chives, with or without a little lemon juice, tamari and olive oil is fantastic;
- Celery stems, and sliced carrot, cucumber or courgette/zucchini are great for dipping into the raw humous, guacamole, paté or seed dips mentioned above – zucchini and celery are relatively easy to grow, whilst cucumbers can require a bit more attention and carrots do best in certain soils (loose/rich/sandy).
- Sprouted green lentils are easy, cheap to produce organically and delicious. Soak them overnight, rinse them once a day and then they're ready in two or three days. I find them simpler and more tasty than many others sprouts. Chick peas are equally easy and delicious, and a great option if you like something to get your teeth into. Alfalfa and radish can be easy too.

A Different Recipe for Salad Success

Take the seeds of a wide range of perennial and self-seeding salad plants – these might be rocket, lettuces, endive/chicory,, kale, tomatoes, perennial spinach, chard, oriental salad greens (Mitsuna or mustard greens), celery, lovage, etc. (see forest garden and permaculture sections for easily grown perennial veg), and add some seeds of edible flowers such as nasturtiums, mallow and calendula. Sprinkle these lightly in appropriate parts of the garden, in large pots or in window boxes. Add water. Add more water according to climatic needs on the days following the day of sowing and then as needed during the growth of the plants. Leave in the sun for 2 to 4 months, and then harvest and eat with some of the other fabulous recipes detailed above.

Sweet Dishes

To encourage a health creating diet, knowing a few good raw sweet dishes is especially useful. However, these dishes should not be used to reinforce unhealthy patterns of behaviour, so beware! For me, the very best sweet dishes are the simplest – fruits on their own!

Devin's Pie (thanks to Devin) - Like Chris's Curry, the legend of Devin's Pie has spread far and wide – many raw food recipe books also have variations of the raw pie! Essential ingredients for this recipe are:

- Dates and almonds are best for the base, sunflower seeds and raisins are good too, although other nuts and seeds can be used.
- Various fruits for the filling, with avocado and banana being great staples for this. Fruits that are 'pretty' either sliced or whole to place on the surface (kiwi, apple, orange, strawberry, grapes, raspberries, etc.).

Mince and mix the dates and almonds (preferably soaked beforehand) in a hand mincer/food processor; sunflower, hemp, walnuts, linseed, etc can also be added. Press this sticky base firmly into a dish (lightly run over the dish with avocado / olive oil before to help when serving). Keep the avocado separate, mixing it with some lemon juice. Blend together all or any of the following: banana, pear, apple, mango, cherimoya, and so on. (Finely ground linseed will thicken the filling or bind the base, but is not essential). Pour this fruit mix into the base first, then spread the mashed / blended avocado layer on top of it.

Slice the 'pretty' fruits finely and lay them on top of the fruit filling to finish off; one or several carefully placed flowers will also add to the 'wow' factor when its brought on to the table. You may need a second one hidden away just in case! Try all sorts of fruit mixes, including blackberry and apple pie or a summer soft fruit pie. Hazel nuts and walnuts can be used as a base also.

Delicious Lemon Pie (thanks to Veronika) - make an almond or other nut base, using dates or raisins to gain the appropriate consistency with the nuts (as per Devin's Pie above). Press the base into a flan dish or a plate (rub oil or avocado lightly on the dish to prevent the base from sticking). Blend together the juice of several lemons with a handful of dates and a little fruit (such as nectarines or peaches), and also include some lemon rind in the blend. Glaze the base with the lemon-date mix, place a layer of sliced fruit on top of this, and then glaze with a second layer of the mix. Absolutely delicious! It's the lemon rind that does it!

Sibila's Sublime Birthday Cake (thanks to Nuria Aragon Castro/Sibila)

Mix together tahini, fresh orange juice, chopped dates, carob powder, some crushed or broken walnut pieces, and then ground sunflower seed and ground linseed to thicken it up. Other nut butters can also be added if you want it even more super rich than it is already. Banana can also be used in the mix. You can have it as a cake or roll it into balls, perhaps rolled in carob powder or finely grated coconut. If it's served as a cake then thin slices of fruit like orange, banana, kiwi or apple can be added to beautify the surface. But remember dishes like this are just for birthdays and special occasions, so don't make them too much of a habit!

My wild guess is that this recipe emerged early in Sibila's raw path, and I think was very much designed for the kids – so it doesn't reflect her own path, aside from recognizing that different people have different needs, including a need for delicious birthday cakes for many.

Raw Chocolate - well, if the western world *is* addicted to chocolate – and it is – then raw chocolate is a way to work with the nature of that reality, as positively as possible. However, some folk appear to have a less than balanced relationship with raw chocolate … but given the addiction, that's not surprising, and raw chocolate has become very popular, playing a big role in widening the interest in eating more raw foods. My own raw chocolate variation adds the option of orange or lemon peel in a mix that is primarily made up of dried seeds and dried fruit:

- ¼ cup raw cacao powder and / or nibs
- ½ cup sunflower and / or pumpkin seeds – almonds or walnuts can also be used
- ¼ linseed / golden flax seed
- 1/4 cup mix of cacao butter and cacao mass, grated (can also be partly coconut butter)
- 1/3 cup raisins / figs / dates

Other possible additions include :
- Orange and / or lemon peel – approx 1 tsp (optional)
- a little Herb Salt (optional)
- Vanilla (optional)
- 1 or 2 Cardomum pods (optional)
- A light dash of chilli powder (optional)

The quantities above are approximate and as with all my own recipes, when making this I always do it by eye and instinct, rather than by measured quantities. For special occasions, or for more chocolate-like raw chocs, swap around the quantities of seeds and cacao butter + mass.

Process: using a good blender, vitamix or masticating juicer, process all the dry ingredients together, then add the dried fruit and grated raw cacao butter / raw cacao mass. Don't over blend as it will get too hot. Remove and form into a block in a dish / container and leave in fridge / cool place for 1-2 hours.

For a super-nutrition version, using superfoods, and want something deliciously nutritious for kids, partners or friends, you can add any or all of the following: goji berries, approx. 20 drops of Marine Minerals' liquid ionic trace minerals or two Marine Minerals Lightning tablets, 1-2 tsp of maca powder, 1-2 tsp mesquite powder, 1-2 tsp green superfoods powder, etc.

Chocolate Brownie (from Holly Paige, www.rawcuisine.co.uk and Funky Raw magazine)
- 4 dates
- 10 dried apricots
- 4 dried figs
- 3 Tbsps sesame seeds
- 15 walnut halves
- 4 tsp raw chocolate powder

Process all the ingredients together until smooth and sticky and shape into bars.
They become firmer and little less sticky after a couple of hours – adding ground linseed will firm them up more.

Lexi's Green Pudding (thanks to Tish)
This is Lexi's pudding in the sense that she loves eating it as well as making it... at least she did when she was five when the first edition of this book was written. It's very simple, and delicious. Just take two avocados, two bananas and the fresh juice of either two oranges or two apples, and blend them all together, dole it out and then eat it. Yum. Oh, yes, and please try to remember to leave some for the kids! To add an extra dimension to the nutritiousness you can add a spoonful of spirulina. To vary the flavour another option is to add a spoonful of carob powder.

Gaura's Sweet Balls (thanks to Gaura)
Soak nuts and seeds (almonds, walnuts, sunflower, etc.) overnight and process or mince them together mainly with dates, raisins or dried figs. Using some unsoaked seeds may help keep the balls firmer. Adding the flesh of sun-dried ripe black olives adds a remarkably delicious bitter-sweet chocolate effect to these sweet balls. Carob also adds to the deliciousness. You can add spices like cinnamon, and even organic fair trade cocoa or carob powder to help soften your taste path on the early transition pathway.

A Cautionary Note On Raw Sweets and Puddings

These sweet dishes can combine many ingredients that often tend not to represent good combining. They taste great to those accustomed to feeding a typical western appetite and therefore have a role, but do not represent the healthiest way to eat. After a while of you will find out if your body reacts differently to them. To me most sweet fruits taste best on their own, and feel better than a complex cake or pudding. It might take you time to adjust of course, but try not to overdo the complex puddings and sweets. Keeping it simple is good.

Generally when it comes to raw food preparation I encourage you to be adventurous, play and experiment in creating beautiful and delicious dishes.

Creating delicious raw meals, whether it's for your daily meals or for a special occasion, is actually much easier than cooking. You can obtain a wider selection of recipes from many sources including Funky Raw (www.funkyraw.com) and Raw Living (www.rawliving.com), with Radiant Children being the single best source for recipes related to children and pregnancy (www.radiantchildren.com). See Appendix 2 for details of other contacts and recipe books.

Some Healthy Options for a 'Mainly Raw' Lifestyle

Breakfast

A breakfast option: oats soaked in spring water with a 'super green' / E3 Live type powder mixed in, with some raisins and / or banana chopped in to sweeten it up.

For kids (or adults): banana mashed with maca powder and flax/omega oil, then add to slightly cooled porridge, with oat milk, goji berries, blueberries and / or a few raisins sprinkled on top. Other chopped fruit can also be added. Or if you've really got to start somewhere much more conventional, half the normal amount of organic cereal (ideally oat-based) or similar, with a little flax / omega / hemp dripped on, then served with blueberries, chopped banana, raisins, gojis and oat milk – it's a start and you can work on things from there!

Practical Working Lunch or School Lunch

Find gluten free crackers or bread (e.g. spelt, rye, etc) used for a salad sandwich, making sure that at least half the meal is raw – this will make a big difference to your after-lunch energy levels if you have a good 'eat more raw' lunch. (If you use cheese, make sure it's goats or sheeps cheese e.g. feta). Include several of the following in each meal.

- Mix of dried fruit and nuts / seeds e.g. brazils, almonds, raisins, figs, pumpkin, sunflower;
- Raw snack bar e.g. Yaoh, etc;   1 or 2 fruits;
- Dehydrated crackers.   Salad mixed with soaked seeds;
- Chunk of cucumber / stick of celery / sticks of carrot;

Dinner

Make a big salad, and eat 1/3 to ½ of it first, and then add steamed / boil potatoes, millet or quinoa to the meal. Try to avoid wheat foods (desert creating in production) e.g. pasta, and rice (rice is greenhouse gas / methane producing in the way it is grown – cattle, and therefore dairy and meat produce, is also a very significant methane / greenhouse gas producer).

PART 11: THE APPENDICES

APPENDIX 1: ABOUT THE AUTHOR

My home is now in West Sussex, England. I've been on the all or mainly raw path since 1994, with 11 of those years raw vegan. From 2000 to 2005, my home was an ecological vegan raw food forest garden project called Ecoforest, in southern Spain, where I lived off grid (no mains electricity, water or sewage) – for those 5 years my dwelling was a large ex-army tent ... But my life hasn't always been like this.

I grew up in deeply middle class west Surrey (England), with a large, beautiful garden to play in. I went from comprehensive school to college to university with no idea what I was doing or where I was going with my life. With a very average Economics & Geography degree, at age 22 I started work for a small steel trading company. My 6 years there provided a great education and confidence building experience, including 3 months working in Los Angeles, USA.

During those years I started waking up - at 24 I started to meditate and explore Buddhist thinking, which I found to be a very practical compassionate philosophy in life. At 28 I quit my 'good job', company car and mortgage, packed up my southern lifestyle (which by that time included anti-nuclear CND demos and Green Party membership) and started an MA in Environmental Planning at the University or Nottingham, ten years after starting my first degree. But this time I knew what I was doing and why.

I focused my studies on sustainability issues, and after 2 years I'd won the course prize with my dissertation, titled 'Planning for Sustainability?' - the question mark is as valid now as it was then! During that time, I also set up a University Green Society with friends, was a student rep on the University Environment Committee and attended local Greenpeace meetings. Life was busy but fun, and much more purposeful. With my MA complete, part-time lecturing followed for the next three years, when I helped set up and deliver a new Green Planning option on my old course, and in 1993 I went to work at the Leicester Environment City project. This was an EU funded project to develop a model approach to working towards urban sustainability – so I was one of the first people in Britain to work on local sustainability strategies and projects as a full-time job.

Whilst in Leicester I saw that the grass-roots was where the main moves towards real sustainability were coming from. And I got involved with permaculture through a life-changing two week permaculture design course in Sept '94 at Turner's Field, Somerset. I also discovered the world of raw food nutrition on that course, when I met Tony Wright, who had already been following that path for 2.1/2 years. Tony has had quite an influence on my life, not only through introducing me to raw food nutrition, but also because of the powerful insights that are now spreading through his ground-breaking book, *Return to the Brain of Eden (Inner Traditions)* – but which at that time were a mass of ideas forming and linking together in his head.[96]

---

[96] Tony Wright and Graham Gynn, *Return to the Brain of Eden*, Inner Traditions (2014). See www.leftinthedark.org.uk/book – you can watch or listen to interviews with Tony via youtube – at the time of writing Tony is working to raise funding for a documentary to critically test and explain his ideas.

I left Leicester in 1995 disillusioned with the political and institutional realities of greenwash amongst senior decision makers and moved down to Devon. With five others, including Tony Wright, Susie Miller (founder of the FRESH network), Dave Austin (now known as Aranya, and one of England's most active permaculture teacher), we established a shared raw food house that became the base for the FRESH Network – the UK's only raw food membership group at the time. The initial group also included Simon and Marijke Shakespeare, who became fantastic leaders in the UK forest schools movement, giving children ecological learning and practical skills in woodland crafts. This house became an information and ad-hoc event centre for the UK's raw food community for 18 months. This was a fascinating, challenging and extraordinary time, that deserves a book in itself – there was far more to it than just the raw food!

As an example, some of the explorations that went on at this time later led to a fully monitored and unique five-day sleep deprivation experiment for Tony and myself with Manchester Metropolitan University, overseen by the respected sports psychologist, Professor Dave Collins. The results are still unique for any supervised sleep deprivation experiment anywhere in the world – over the 5 days on average we experienced *improved* dexterity, physical agility and mental acuity, without any stimulants and with us just eating *our* normal (raw) diet. Why? Well one fact is that it's the only such experiment to have ever involved long term raw fooders - so that has a lot to do with the unique results – our normal diet was 100% raw, with about 70% fruit. You can read more about this and many other fascinating issues in Tony Wright's *Return to the Brain of Eden*. Tony went on to break the world staying awake record some years later – just over 11 days awake, carrying out coherent interviews at the point when the record was broken!

Around that time, I also connected up with the Plants for a Future project, met Robert Hart for the first time, and did lots of writing and personal research on a whole range of issues (particularly sustainability issues and their relationship to human social patterns, economic patterns, patterns of civilization and patterns of thinking, understanding/misunderstanding, perception expressed through our consciousness, etc.). I also ran a series of local permaculture courses with Simon Shakespeare and we set up a local permaculture network – The Exe Valley Permaculture Network, and hosted my first 12 day permaculture design certificate course (one student on that course was Aranya). I then had some interesting times including six months living at Turner's Field, near Glastonbury, with my good friend (Ann) Morgan and an enigmatic northern Irish chap called Louis. I then visited possibly the most extraordinary place and people I have ever met – Tiaia in western Eire, an awesomely beautiful, barefoot, place of 'ecotarian' paradise gardening, and a universe in itself, rooted in the deepest understanding and experience of nature I've lived within. Nine months barefoot followed this visit ... which was fantastically enlivening and not difficult most of the time (although I wasn't doing any conventional work at that time!). The barefoot phase came to a close because in this culture I found that, outside of community situations, it can be tiring living in ways that don't fit the norm. It was also heading for winter and I had started regularly visiting Robert Hart, travelling by motorbike... which didn't suit bare feet!

It was the winter before Robert died, and I was trying to help him produce the book he so desperately wanted to write – which became very difficult because of my penniless circumstances, my stretched commitments elsewhere, and because of Robert's variable health. One day I hope to produce some more direct results of that friendship, as a book.

From 1998 to 2000 two things happened. Firstly, I started reconnecting with the establishment world of sustainability. And secondly, on the grass roots side, with a diverse group of a dozen people I helped propose and establish Ecoforest - an ecological vegan raw food community and eco-education project in Spain. In 1999 I set up a community enterprise called Somerset Sustainable Housing with my highly skilled and motivated timber framer friend, Jim Blackburn (who formed The Timber Frame Company Ltd around that time), and completed The Somerset Sustainable Housing Study. And as a result of this work, in 2000 I was employed for 6 months by South Somerset District Council and Somerset County Council, to design and implement the pioneering South Somerset Sustainable Construction Strategy, which lead to the establishment of the Somerset Trust for Sustainable Development – renamed Ecos Trust in 2007.

After some early struggles, thanks to the persistence and hard work over the years of its first manager, subsequent Director, staff and trustees, STSD flourished for years as Ecos Trust (www.ecostrust.org.uk), as a training and educational organisation, consultancy, and ethical community-based developer (Ecos Homes) that *only* undertook pioneering high quality and affordable sustainable housing and construction projects. The Trust's mission was 'to make sustainable construction the norm, rather than the exception'. I relinquished my part-time role as Planning & Research Director of the Trust in 2003.

My role with the Trust became smaller because from 2001 I was spending most of my time at Ecoforest, which went well for several years, but then became more focused on visitors' needs than the residents' needs – and I became a little stuck there. Ecoforest worked very well for many visitors, with over 600 people staying there between 2000 and 2005, for periods of time between a day and a year – most stayed for at least a week, and many for more than a month. It was a place that changed many lives, because whilst you were there you were in a place and amongst people where *the raw food lifestyle was normal for 365 days of the year*, and not different. That experience was very powerful for many people, and is not something that can be recreated on a raw food retreat or food preparation class. It was also not about making money – there were financial aspects of course, but its main focus was affordability. The low impact living, off grid and close to nature aspect of Ecoforest was also a vital part of the experience – in many ways what we were doing at Ecoforest was creating a place that provided the chance to live the lifestyle described in Gordon Kennedy's great book, *Children of the Sun*.

A whole host of amazing people spent time at Ecoforest, and went on to do amazing things in the healthy living, raw food and permaculture movements, from Rob of Funky Raw, to Diana Store (rawsuperfoods.com) and Laura de Nooijer (Lovechock) in the Netherlands, to Paulo Mellett (who helped establish Lush cosmetics' Slush Fund), to Veronika Poola (Jaramuza Retreats), to Henri Dobson (who helped found London's annual Festival of Life) and Chris Kennett (of veggiepower.co.uk and for many years also involved in London's Festival of Life) ... to name but a few – there were many, many more.

Eventually in summer 2005 I returned to England's green landscape, and life has evolved since then with family, home and fatherhood. For 7 years until 2012, I lived in a well-established community in West Sussex (southern England, established 1972), which is home to about 65 people in 27 homes, with 3 community buildings, and a wood chip fuelled community heating system. The community has Anthroposophical roots, founded around the ideas of Rudolf Steiner, an Austrian philosopher who founded biodynamic agriculture and Waldorf education. I left the community in 2012, now living close by, gradually eco-retrofitting my small house.

My primary work is as a sustainability consultant, with a particular focus on pioneering and innovative sustainability projects and strategies, especially in relation to sustainable building skills, training and education. I also teach permaculture courses, and aim to start providing 'Real Health' courses in the future, based on a concept developed with Dr Nichol Clarke.

Great change and great diversity in my life has included going from being barefoot to wearing a suit 'n' tie as a consultant to various Councils within one year (1999 - 2000); from living in a tent off-grid on a Spanish hillside to initiating a project with Britain's largest county council 6 months later (2005), which led to a unique £5mn+ centre for sustainable building training in north Kent with the most comprehensive regional sustainable building training programme in the country. These have been interesting reality shifts. Both were very positive experiences, although the mainstream consultancy work is a little harder and less fun than the former because of the resistance to real, positive change that is deeply embedded across all sectors in Britain. But it shows that such things are possible. More recently I've co-written the UK's first accredited sustainable building qualifications, mainly working voluntarily for a not-for-profit (Green Gauge Trust) because government and industry were too ill-informed and unaware to put these in place or realize they are vital if we are to create low energy, low carbon buildings with a construction, building design, property and housing workforce of around 2 million people. So with a handful of others we've just got on and did it ourselves, knowing it needs to be done. Since 2012 I've been working as Education Development Manager for the Bay Trust, which runs Europe's lowest impact conference and events venue (the Pines Calyx) and a residential outdoor learning centre, Rippledown, which caters for school groups, with over 2000 children experiencing the wonderful 'Rippledown effect' each year – I have also helped develop and deliver Britain's first training to close 'the performance gap' in buildings, working with the Good Homes Alliance.

So since Sept 1994 I have maintained a 90-100% raw diet, with 10 years of being 100% raw vegan. I was vegan from 1991 to 2005, and have been vegetarian since 1988. Since the winter of '94-5 I have eaten 1 cooked meal (a curry, as an experiment with Aranya back in about '98, which was horrible!) and have tasted two small pieces of bread since '94 (it tasted salty, stodgy, lifeless and generally weird), and have enjoyed excellent health, well above average, and often been very active with people often thinking I am five to ten years younger than my age.

However, at times in my raw journey I have had a patchy and difficult relationship with the one addictive drug that has most strongly influenced my life – namely coffee! (Yes, ok, the drug is caffeine, I know.) Man! It's only when you come off such things that you realise how powerful an effect these highly profitable, legal drugs have (sugar, alcohol and nicotine being the three other obvious ones). This kind of realisation often happens when your eyes first open! For me, coffee has been very strongly associated with work, sitting at a PC or going to meetings, doing work that I felt was important (often with few if any others able or willing to do it), but which I often did not really want to be doing. Coffee is effective in shutting down my sensitivities whilst living in a world that often feels harsh, destructive and uncaring – as well as more than a little insane, when you've had the chance to step back from 'normality' to see it for what it is. This may be useful as a survival strategy, but caffeine definitely has a harsh effect on one's emotions and nervous system, and its addictive quality has helped me maintain my inner conflict about using it. On coffee I am a different person – not my true self, and left feeling more 'acid' and stressed when its initial effects wear off. So whilst I had no desire to slip back into plates and pans of cooked food, for varying lengths of time I have swum around in mugs and jugs of coffee for far too long! I've had lengthy periods off coffee – but when on it, it has kept me working in areas that are essentially positive and still feel hugely important, but which are dealing with the symptoms and not the underlying causes of ill-health and an unsustainable culture, economy and lifestyle.

Most of these years, having discovered raw food and the power of permaculture back in '94, I have lived in places where I could quickly create a good salad garden, or where one already existed – this has been really important. Placing a few seeds and a special selection of perennials in the ground has a wonderful effect – it creates food! So I enjoyed the delights of a vibrant and varied fresh-picked home grown and wild green salad on the vast majority of evenings from '94 to 2005, as well as very regularly since then, with the joys of Turner's Field and Tiaia salads being the peaks of that particular experience! Getting those really vibrant greens in almost every day has been 'vital'. As much as anything else, I feel that consistently eating plenty of fresh greens has been important in sustaining my health.

Over the years I have written down my thoughts about all these issues which are close to my heart, and have self-published these thoughts in the books *The Earth Dwellers Guide to Sustainability* and *Sustainability, Consciousness and Climate Change*.[97] As I've worked in the sustainability field for so long, usually in pioneering areas, I have to say that there is not much hard evidence of meaningful action to convince me that as a society we will respond sufficiently and quickly enough to the challenges of climate change, species loss and ecosystems devastation, and so much more. But you never know, anything's possible!

And as for this book, well it's an outcome of all those experiences, and it results as much from the people I've met along the way, their work and the inspiration they have provided, as it does from my own efforts. So I thank you all, my friends, and I hope that this book does as much good for the reader as the experiences I've described above have done for the writer!

To sum up my experience of the food-diet-lifestyle issue – I have definitely felt my best, on a consistent basis, when I was 100% raw vegan over a significant period of time. At the same time, I recognize that's not a realistic starting point or objective for many people in the world we live in. It's also not where I am at now, although that's the result of compromise, circumstance and a balance of choices which isn't always easy. And I do expect to go forward to where I have been in the past at some time in my life – in other words, back to being fully raw but in a different way, with more experience and understanding.

My last words are, have fun and don't be afraid to adventure with your life folks – I can tell you from experience that living a healthier and much more sustainable life can be a whole lot of fun and it's a great way to learn about yourself and the vibrant world we are part of! And, whether it's health, diet, lifestyle.

Steve Charter, 2016

---

[97] Available via www.lulu.com – and hopefully available on Amazon and from other sources by the time you read this !

APPENDIX 2: CONTACTS, RESOURCES AND INFORMATION

RAW FOOD AND NATURAL HEALTH CONTACTS AND INFORMATION
LIVING/RAW FOODS NETWORKS, ORGANISATIONS and ONLINE SHOPS
In the UK
- Funky Raw at www.funkyraw.com: great magazine, events and on-line shop;
- Eat More Raw at www.eatmoreraw.org;
- Raw Reform (Angela Stokes) at www.rawreform.co.uk - particularly good for successful, inspiring and sustained weight-loss through healthy eating;
- Detox Your World/Shazzie at www.detoxyourworld.com and www.shazzie.com;
- Raw Living at www.rawliving.co.uk workshops and on-line shop run by Kate Wood author of *Eat Smart, Eat Raw* and *Raw Living* – see books section below for full references;
- Karen Knowler's site at www.therawfoordcoach.com – for both raw coaching and raw business coaching – www.karenknowler.com;
- The FRESH Network: Web: www.fresh-network.com - *Get Fresh!* mag, on-line shop, etc;
- Elaine Bruce at www.livingfoods.co.uk – living foods education, training and information;
- Mike Nash at www.aggressivehealth.co.uk – for blokes keen on strength and fitness;
- Festival of Life at www.festivaloflife.net, great annual event in London and web-resource;
- *Nature's First Law* and David Wolfe, CA. – possibly the world's most dynamic, active and effective raw food advocate and motivational speaker in the last 10-15 years - www.rawfood.com and www.davidwolfe.com
- Hippocrates Health Institute, Dr Brian Clement & Anne-Marie Clement - http://www.hippocratesinst.org/
- *Vibance* e-magazine. Web: www.livingnutrition.com – edited by David Klein;
- Gabriel Cousens / Tree of Life Centre, AZ – an advanced and effective approach with a medical background and a spiritual dimension - www.treeoflife.nu
- Dr Douglas Graham, President of Healthful Living International - an international authority on athletic performance and living foods nutrition. Web: www.doctorgraham.cc
- Frederic Paténaude: www.fredericpatenaude.com and online mag Pure Health & Nutrition;
- Healthful Living International - Doug Graham, Dave Klein, Dr Vivian Vetrano, Prof. Roz Gruben and others – combined knowledge & experience -: www.healthfullivingintl.org
- Paul Nison, New York, NY – author of *The Raw Life & Raw Knowledge* - www.rawlife.com
- Cherie Soria and *Living Light International* at www.rawfoodchef.com
- Raw Family, www.rawfamily.com – the Boutenko family's much visited website;
- Dr Joel Robbins, medical practitioner with outstanding CDs – the best general introduction I've found yet - available from www.drdonnavice.com/drobbins/index.php

OTHER INTERNATIONAL RAW FOODS CONTACTS
- *Raw Super Foods*, Amsterdam/Nederlands, coordinated by Diana Store – www.rawsuperfoods.com - excellent information, courses and retreats in Amsterdam and around Europe, products and a weekly stall at Amsterdam's organic Noordermarkt;

- *Fruitarian Info* – http://www.fruitarian.info
- *Die Wurzel* – the leading network, congresses and magazine, in Germany (Wurzel-Gesundheitsforum) - www.die-wurzel.de
- Nuria Aragon Castro, Spain – pursuing a spiritual path (Sant Mat), of which vegetarian whole raw foods is just one part, author of several inspiring books in Spanish (published by Mandala Ediciones) on simple natural living - www.nuriaaragoncastro.com
- Cana Dulce, southern Spain – a truly wonderful place for permaculture/forest garden and yoga courses, natural hygiene, raw and eco-living at www.permacutluracanadulce.org

OTHER LIVING/RAW FOOD READING

- *Raw Secrets*, by Frederic Paténaude, (Raw Vegan, 2002) recommended for an honest handbook on the pros & cons of raw life - and *Sunfood Cuisine*, (Nature's First Law, 2002).
- Books by Dr Douglas Graham: *Nutrition and Athletic Performance* (FoodnSport, 2008) is excellent, simple and clear, focused on fitness, sport and health – also *Grain Damage*, FoodnSport (2005) and *The New High Energy Diet Recipe Guide*, FoodnSport (2007).
- *Raw Life* (2000) and *Raw Knowledge* (2003) both self-published by Paul Nison – these books make inspiring and practical reading.
- *The Sunfood Diet Success System* (True North Productions, 1999) by David Wolfe – continuing to have a huge impact - also *Eating For Beauty* (North Atlantic Books, 2008), and *Nature's First Law* (True North Productions, 1998), with Steven Arlin and RC Dini.
- *Detox Your World* (Raw Creation, 2003) by Shazzie, available from www.detoxyourworld.com for a nurturing approach;
- *Raw Reform* e-book and *Raw Emotions*, Monarch Publishing (2009) by Angela Stokes – excellent on raw nutrition, weight-loss, and the emotional aspect: www.rawreform.co.uk
- *Naked Chocolate*, North Atlantic Books (2008) by David Wolfe and Shazzie.
- *Intuitive Eating* by Susie Miller & Karen Knowler, (The Women's Press, 2000).
- *Conscious Eating*, North Atlantic Books (2004) and *Rainbow Green Live Food Cuisine*, North Atlantic Books (2003) by Dr Gabriel Cousens – from an ayurvedic perspective;
- *Eat Smart Eat Raw*, Grub Street (2002) and *Raw Living*, Grub Street (2007) by Kate Wood, good introductions and recipe books – from www.rawliving.co.uk
- *12 Steps to Raw*, Raw Family Publishing (2001) by Victoria Boutenko, adapted from the world renowned and highly successful addiction-breaking '12 step program';
- *Fats That Kill, Fats That Heal*, Alive Books (1993) by Dr Udo Erasmus - book and CD;
- *Dick Gregory's Natural Diet for Folks Who Eat: Cookin' With Mother nature*, by Dick Gregory et al, HarperPerennial (1974) – a great raw starter with humour and feeling.
- *The New Raw Energy* by Leslie and Susannah Kenton, Vermilion, London, 1994;
- *Health Through Nutrition* and *Attitudes to Health* CDs by Dr. Joel Robbins. – brilliantly presented information and advice – from www.drdonnavice.com/drobbins/index.php
- *Children of the Sun*, Nivaria Press (1998) by Gordon Kennedy – a wonderful book about the people of the raw and natural health movement and its European and US origins.
- Franz Konz, the German raw food 'bible' *Der Grosse Gesundheits*, Univertas Verlag (1998)

- *The Sprouters Handbook* (Edward Kearney) and *Sprouting in the UK* (Sally Holloway)
- Sibila's (Nuria Aragon Castro) first book: *Vida Libre y Natural: en el sendero de la sencillez y el amor* (Free and Natural Life: on the trail of simplicity and love) includes chapters on the simple raw vegan nutrition, home education, not vaccinating, and other fascinating elements 'on the pathway of a free and natural life' (Mandala Ediciones, Madrid, 2002. ISBN 84 95052 82 0) – also *Observando a la Vida, Mistica en la Vida Diaria, Sentimientos dibujos y reflexiones* and *Vivir sin Cole* – see www.nuriaaragoncastro.com
- *Comiendo Pura Vida*, Apro (2002) by Rodrigo Crespo Apéstegui, an excellent Spanish introduction, including recipes by Cherie Soria (ISBN 9977-05-050-3)
- Jose Manuel Casada Sierra – *Las Frutas, Nuestro Alimento Ideal* (Madrid, 2007) - excellent Spanish raw book, with recipes and information. ISBN 84 88722 095.

RAW RECIPE BOOKS

There are so many raw recipe books these days that I am not listing any here, although most of the above books include recipes. Beware of recipes which look great, no doubt taste fantasic, but which really are not realistic in terms of time to prepare and complexity, as part of a day-to-day 'eat more raw' diet.

RAW PARENTING

Information sources and books to help parents and children are growing all the time now – many are designed to help with less than 100% raw lifestyles and transitioning, whilst some focus on a 100% raw lifestyle. Some of the excellent resources that are now available include:
- The Boutenko Family (US) – and *Raw Family*: a true story of awakening. Web: www.rawfamily.com
- *Evie's Kitchen: Raising an Ecstatic Child*, Raw Creation (2008) by Shazzie
- *Raw Kids* by Cheryl Stoykoff – transitioning kids to a raw food diet. Web: www.livingspiritfoundation.org
- *The Mother Magazine*: www.themothermagazine.co.uk - excellent on natural mothering, including raw foods section.
- *Get Fresh* magazine, Fresh Network UK has a regular raw parenting column.
- *The Continuum Concept* by Jean Liedloff, Perseus Books - an important book, when translated to the current cultural context, although not about diet or nutrition.

SOME OF THE ON-LINE RAW STORES AND RESOURCES

For books, foods (particularly superfoods), equipment and more: #
www.funkyraw.com
www.fresh-network.com
www.rawsuperfoods.com
www.detoxyourworld.com
www.rawreform.com
www.rawfood.com
www.rawliving.com
www.tree-harvest.com
www.livingnutrition.com

These days there's obviously tons of resources available on the internet, with youtube, numerous Facebook groups, and many other resources making the entry into the world of raw food nutrition, and healthy living in general, so much more direct than it was 20 years ago.

OTHER CONTACTS FOR ELEMENTS OF WHOLE HEALTH

Meditation: Transcendental Meditation (www.meditationtrust.com for affordable courses) and Vipassana can be found through the internet, as can the Federation of Western Buddhists.

Yoga and Tai Chi: *The Five Tibetans*, Christopher Kilham (Healing Arts Press, 1994). Tons of books on yoga and tai chi – best to find a teacher, take a course, and continue the practice yourself regularly either independently or with a local group.

Ki Aikido: Enquiries verbally or via www.Ki-aikido.net (USA) or www.Kifedgb.force9.co.uk (UK) will find a local or regional teacher, or course.

Artistic and creative endeavours: many books and courses help you express your creative side in a healthy and positive way – *The Artist's Way*, Pan Books (1997) by Julia Cameron and *The Healing Voice*, Element Books (1999) by Paul Newham are examples.

Community, group work and communication: *Creating Harmony* edited by Hildur Jackson (Permenant Publications, 1999) on the realities of community living. *Communities* magazine - http://www.ic.org/communities-magazine-home/ - is excellent, for North America. In the UK and Europe; *Diggers and Dreamers!* (Diggers and Dreamers Publications, 2008) and the *Eurotopia* (http://www.eurotopia.de) are good directories of intentional communities available via www.green-shopping.co.uk, as is *Non Violent Communication* (Puddle Dancer Press, 2003) – also via www.cnvc.org and www.LifeResouces.co.uk For tons of relevant information for communities seeking to transition to sustainability – www.transitiontowns.org

PERMACULTURE INFORMATION, NETWORKS AND ORGANISATIONS

- UK Pc Association – address: BCM Permaculture Association, London WC1N 3XX. Tel: 01654 712 188. Email: office@permaculture.org.uk Web: www.permaculture.org.uk
- Permaculture Magazine – just excellent - Permanent Publications: The Sustainability Centre, East Meon, Hampshire GU32 1HR. - www.permaculture.co.uk
- Geoff Lawton, probably the world's most active permaculture educator – with excellent online information and courses available - http://geofflawton.com/
- Open Permaculture – another very active online source of courses and information - https://www.openpermaculture.com/
- Aranya's permaculture website - http://www.learnpermaculture.com/
- Agroforestry Research Trust, Dartington, Devon – excellent books, DVD, research and demonstration gardens – www.agroforestry.co.uk
- Plants For A Future: PFAF, Research Centre and Demonstration - Web:www.pfaf.org
- VON (Vegan Organic Network): Web: www.veganorganic.net
- For courses see www.permaculture.org.uk list of courses and events, look in *Permaculture Magazine* or visit Designed Visions at www.designedvisions.com
- Permaculture Design Magazine: P.O. Box 60669, Sunnyvale, CA 94088 USA. Web: http://permaculturedesignmagazine.com/

- *American Permaculture Directory*: Email:jwirwin@permaculture.net
- Earthaven Ecovillage: Black Mountain, NC 28711. Web: www.earthaven.org
- Permaculture Institute USA: New Mexico. Email: pci@permaculture-inst.org
- Central Rocky Mountain Permaculture Institute: Web: www.crmpi.org
- Mountain Gardens (and Permaculture Seed and Plant Exchange), 546 Shuford Creek Road, Burnsville, NC 28714. USA. www.mountaingardensherbs.com
- Formidable Vegetable Sound System – http://formidablevegetable.com.au/ - for great and inspiring permaculture music!

AUSTRALIA:

- Djanburg Gardens and Permaculture College Australia: Nimbin, NSW. Email: permed@nor.cor.au Web: www.earthwise.org.au
- Permaculture Research Institute: www.permaculture.org.au - international non-profit charitable organization working with communities worldwide to expand knowledge and practice using the whole-systems approach of Permaculture Design;
- SEED International: 50 Crystal Waters, Kilroy Lane, Conondale, QLD 4552. Email: info@permaculture.au.com Web: www.permaculture.au.com
- David Holmgren, Holmgren Design Services: www.holmgren.com.au

EXCELLENT TEMPERATE CLIMATE RESOURCES *(E.G. FOR EUROPE AND N AMERICA)*

- *Agroforestry News*: Agroforestry Research Trust, 46 Hunters Moon, Dartington, Totnes, Devon TQ9 6JT – UK based, invaluable for temperate areas: www.agroforestry.co.uk
- Plants for a Future at www.pfaf.org – online database;
- *Growing Green International*: Vegan Organic Network, www.veganorganic.net – international magazine on vegan organic agriculture, horticulture and permaculture.

PERMACULTURE WEBSITES

www.permaculture.org.uk   www.permaculture.co.uk   http://www.permacultureglobal.com/
www.gaiauniversity.org   www.crmpi.org   www.earthhaven.org
www.gaia.org.ar   www.permaculture.org.au   www.permacultureactivist.net
www.permaculture.au.com   www.permaculture.net   www.permacultureinstitute.com
www.permaculture.org.nz   www.holmgren.com.au   www.spiralseed.co.uk
www.aranyagardens.co.uk   www.designedvisions.com   www.permaculturacanadulce.org
www.permacultura-es.org   www.permakultur-akademie.de

Again, tons of fantastic resources are available on the 'net, with youtube films, on-line courses, Facebook groups, and many other resources making the permaculture world highly accessible.

PUBLISHERS AND MAIL ORDER BOOK SUPPLIERS

- www.permaculture.co.uk and www.green-shopping.co.uk - Permanent Publications site.
- www.chelseagreen.com – Chelsea Green Publishing – US publishers.

- www.tagari.com – publisher's of Bill Mollison's books.
- www.eco-logicbooks.com - in the UK

PERMACULTURE READING

A huge range of useful books is available by mail order from Permanent Publications (UK), all described in their excellent catalogue *The Green Shopping Catalogue* (www.green-shopping.co.uk), and from Chelsea Green (USA) – addresses as above – the best introductory books for any climate:
- *An Introduction to Permaculture* (228 pages), Bill Mollison and Reny Mia Sley, Tagari Press (1998), and *Permaculture: A Designers' Manual*, Tagari (1988; 576 pages), by Bill Mollison which is the 'bible' of the permaculture movement.
- *The Earthcare Manual* (2004), *How To Make A Forest Garden (1996)* and *Permaculture In A Nutshell* (1993) all by Patrick Whitefield, and all published by Permanent Publications – practical, packed with information, by Britain's leading permaculture teacher.
- *The Basics of Permaculture Design* by Ross Mars, Permanent Publications (2005) – an accessible and practical book.
- *Forest Gardening* (Green Books, 1996) is THE text book on the subject, and *Beyond The Forest Garden* (Gaia Books, 1996) for the background philosophy, both by Robert Hart.
- *Creating a Forest Garden,* Martin Crawford, Agroforestry Research Trust (2010) and excellent *A Year in a Forest Garden* DVD
- *Designing and Maintaining Your Edible Landscape* by Robert Kourik, Metamorphic Press (1986) – does not cover permaculture design, but great for the gardening side of pc.
- *Permaculture Design: a step by step guide* by Aranya, Permanent Publications (2012) – the first authoritative guide to the process and tools of permaculture design, to be used as a practical handbook (rather than for a cover-to-cover read).

Some other excellent books are:
- *Food For Free* by Richard Mabey, Collins (2007), or *Wild Food* by Roger Philips, Pan Books (1983).
- *How To Grow More Vegetables: Than you ever thought possible on less land than you can imagine* by John Jeavons, Ten Speed Press (1995) – the title says it all!
- *Plants For A Future* by Ken Fern, Permanent Publications (2000) – just superb.
- *Permaculture Plants* by Jeff Nugent & Julia Boniface, Chelsea Green (2009) – excellent for Mediterranean/sub-tropical and tropical climates.
- *The Permaculture Garden* (2008) and *The Permaculture Way* (2008) by Graham Bell, Permanent Publications – for an excellent overall perspective.
- *Permaculture: a beginners guide*, by Graham Burnett, Spiralseed (2008), an excellent and simple illustrated guide – available from www.spiralseed.co.uk;

SEED AND PLANT SUPPLIERS

Good sources for good seed, plant and tree suppliers are up-to-date copies of *Permaculture Magazine* (UK), or *Permaculture Activist* (USA) – or by web searches for organic seeds and permaculture plants:
- The Agroforestry Research Trust (UK, and will supply to many other countries) – supplying seeds and plants – absolutely excellent and large range from trees, to shrubs, to ground cover plants and climbers: 46 Hunters Moon, Dartington, Totnes, Devon TQ9 6JT, UK. Web: www.agroforestry.co.uk
- Chase Organics – www.chaseorganics.co.uk
- Seed Savers Exchange - http://www.seedsavers.org

THE FOOD SYSTEM, ECONOMY, SUSTAINABILITY & THE MEDICAL SYSTEM

- *Bringing The Food Economy Home* by Norberg-Hodge, Merrifield and Gorelick (Zed Books, 2002) – local alternatives to global agri-business and the wholesale economic, social and environmental destruction it wreaks.
- *The Food System* by Tansey and Worsley (Earthscan, 1995) is an excellent book on the realities of the food sytem and economy from global to local level.
- *Dead Doctors Don't Lie* by Dr Joel Wallach (book and CD), Legacy Communications (1999) provides an apparently objective perspective on the effectiveness (or lack of it) of the modern western medical system, and its overall health impacts, costs, etc.
- *The China Study* by T Colin Campbell, Be Bella (2006) – subtitled: *The most comprehensive study of nutrition ever conducted and the stratlingimplications for diet, weight loss and long term health* – says it all.
- *Feeding People Is Easy* by Colin Tudge, Pari Publishind (2007) – a straight-forward analysis of why the current industrial agriculture system is fundamentally unsustainable, with practical suggestions as to what is needed in response.

APPENDIX 3: AN OUTLINE FOR ESTABLISHING A FOREST GARDEN

TEMPERATE CLIMATES

The following table gives an *indication* of stacking in time and space, primarily *using perennial plants* to achieve an all year raw harvest with a 'skeleton' forest garden system in a temperate climate. Actual seasons will vary according to the varieties chosen, as well as the climate you are in and the micro-climate you can create or take advantage of to extend the season. The Agroforestry Research Trust and Plants for a Future in the UK, and the various seed saving / plant exchanges in the US which are listed in the Appendices section supply an extensive variety of less common fruits which can extend your all year harvest significantly. They and others listed in the Appendices section also supply a very wide variety of salad plants.

Sprouting dried legumes and pulses allows an all year round cheap addition to salads that can be easily obtained organic. Using lettuces planted in succession, as well various annuals in the cabbage family and oriental green vegetables can extend the winter vegetables significantly. Some of these plants will be able to self-seed very successfully, as will celery.

The information above and in the following pages will help you create an all-year round food producing system. A good start is to select around 20 to 30 perennial salad plants in the herbaceous and ground cover sections for an all year salad garden – perennial kale, broccoli and onions, perpetual spinach and peltaria/garlic cress are highly recommended as core elements in your salad system.

More information is provided for apples and pears as they are most likely to form the skeleton around which a temperate forest garden is created. The lists of plants are by no means exclusive, and much good information on herbaceous plants in general, including self-seeders, 'cut and come again' plants and other salad plants is contained in various permaculture books; the book *Plants For A Future* by Ken Fern and Martin Crawford's *Creating a Forest Garden* being particularly superb references.

For very accessible information, Alys Folwer's books and information on the internet are a really practical and straight-forward general source of information on veg growing, salads and herbs.

	Jan-April	May-June	July-Aug	Sept-Oct	Nov-Dec
Canopy	Stored apples and pears, dried fruits & nuts.	Dried fruits and nuts.	Apples, Plums, Gages. Mulberry, Cherry Plum,	Apples, Pears, Plums. Walnut, Chestnut, Butternuts, Shagbark Hickory, American Oaks, Pine-nuts.	Apples, Pears, Nepalese and Willow-leaved Buckthorn (Hippophae Rhamnoides/ Salicifolia), Persimmon.
Understorey	Hawthorn leaves.	Juneberry. Lime tree leaves.	Peach, Apricot, Brown Turkey Fig.	Oregon grape (Mahonia aquifolium / repens). Crab Apple, edible Rowan and Hawthorns. Hazel/Filbert.	Medlar.
Climbers			Blackberry.	Siberian kiwi, Romanus Rosehips, Grapes	
Shrub		Eleagnus, Gooseberry, Saltbush.	Raspberry (early), Red/White Currants, Loganberry, Tayberry, Gooseberry, Blackcurrants, Japanese Wineberry, Saltbush.	Raspberry (late), Chinese dogwood, Thimbleberry, Salmonberry, Saltbush.	
Herbaceous	Alexanders	Rocket, Samphire, Polish Sorrel, Tree onions, Welsh onions, Mallow, Horseradish, Good King Henry, Dandelions, Fennel, Dill, Sweet Cicely, Lovage, Campanulas, Tomatoes (self-seeded). Sweet Cicely, Alpine Dock, Turkish rocket.			
	Chives, Perennial Kale, Perennial spinach, Perennial Broccoli, Perennial onions and garlic (Welsh onion, Tree onion, Everlasting onion, Garlic chives, Serpent garlic).				
	Wild garlic/ Ransoms, Jack-by-the-Hedge.			oriental greens e.g. mizuna, Chinese cabbage, leaf mustards, pak choi,	
Ground-cover	Corn salad		Clovers		Corn salad
Root-crops	Beetroot, Parsnip, Carrot.			Beetroot, Parsnip, Carrot, Turnips, Swede, Celeriac, Kohl Rabi	

Apples - are the most important fruit for the temperate climate as they are amongst the hardiest fruit and can be stored for use all year. Apples can be grown as:
- Standards: plant 4.6-6m (15-20ft) apart;
- Bush trees: plant 2.4-3m (8-10 ft) apart;
- Cordons: plant 1.2m (4ft) apart at 45 degree angle to restrict sap flow and growth;
- Dwarf Pyramids: plant 1.8-2.1m (6-7ft) apart, produce most fruit in the shortest time.

Dwarf trees bear fruit rather than produce wood, and come more quickly to heavy fruit bearing. Trees on dwarfing root-stock need careful staking as they do not produce such strong roots. A strong stake is needed approx. 0.3m (1ft) from the roots, at a slight angle, with the bark protected from rubbing against the stake in windy weather.

Apples need a soil with humus for moisture retention for the fruit to make a good size. Grass needs suppressing with mulch around the tree when planted to reduce competition for nutrients. Most apples need other varieties for pollination i.e. they do not set fruit with pollen from their own variety. A mix of varieties is usually important, matched up for whether they are early / mid / late flowering varieties, with edible crab-apples being excellent all-round pollinators.

Pears - originate from a warmer climate than apples, so require more warmth to ripen properly – hence their use particularly in walled gardens. They can be grown in standard, bush, pyramid or cordon forms, and are often best grown in Espalier form along walls, or trained along strong guides. Pruning, pollination and culture is similar to apples.

Plums and Gages – need carefully selection and siting, particularly for warmth.

Other Fruit (see particularly *Plants for a Future* and *Agroforestry Research Trust*)
Sea buckthorn - *Hippophae salicifolia* or *Rhamnoides* – a superfood, and medicinally powerful; Edible hawthorns, *Crataegus* – various varieties, many with excellent and surprising fruits. Other delicious fruit include: medlar; edible rowan; cherry;
Warmth and sun loving fruit and nuts (with shelter from wind): Peaches, apricots, mulberry, American persimmon, brown turkey fig, whitebeam, almonds;

Nuts
Walnut: buccaneer/broadview, chestnut: *Castenea mollissima/cretana*, butternuts, shagbark hickory, American oaks, pine nuts: stone pine/Swiss arola pine/Mexican nut-pine

Edible Tree Leaves - Lime, *Ginkgo biloba* (for circulation and brain health), hawthorn leaves;

FRUITING CLIMBERS - Blackberry (wild and thornless varieties), loganberry, tayberry; Siberian kiwi, NZ kiwi, Romanus rosehips - Grape: brant vine/*Vitis coignitiae*/strawberry grape

UNDERSTOREY TREES - Shade tolerants include: medlar, juneberry, lime tree leaves, oregon grape (*Mahonia aquifolium/repens*), hazel/filbert, crab apples

SHRUBS - *Good shade tolerant bushes and cane fruit:* Gooseberry~, loganberry~, Japanese wineberry~, *Eleagnus, Rosa rugosa*, raspberry, red/white currants, autumn raspberry, mulberry, blackcurrants, Chinese dogwood, thimbleberry, salmonberry
On acid soils, or in containers: blueberry, cowberry, dewberry;
Saltbush/*Atriplex halimus*.
See also: Plants for a Future and Agroforestry Research Trust;

HERBACEOUS LEVEL - See *Creating a Forest Garden* (by Martin Crawford), *How to Make a Forest Garden* (by Patrick Whitefield), *Forest Gardening* (by Robert Hart), *Plants for a Future* (book or website), Agroforestry Research Trust (website). For those interested in a historical perspective and traditional English salad plants also see: *John Evelyn's Acetaria*: a discourse on sallets (first pub'd 1699, facsimile copies printed more recently) for a superb range of herbal 'sallet' plants. **All Year Round Herbaceous Salad Leaves Or Available During The Winter, including some wild plants** - Three-cornered leek, spinach beet, *Campanula versiculor*, salad burnet, Turkish rocket, alexanders, dandelions, perennial kale, perennial broccoli, hedge garlic, daffodil garlic, wild garlic, Welsh onions, perennial onion, chives, fennel, sweet cicely, alpine dock, lovage, Good King Henry, Polish sorrel, samphire, mitsuba, corn salad, horseradish, tree onions, Welsh onions, landcress, ribbed plantain.

GROUND COVER - All Year Round Ground Cover Salad Leaves Or Available During The Winter - *Peltaria alliacea, Richardia picroides*, sorrel/*Rumex acetosa*, miner's lettuce, ground ivy, hairy bittercress, pink purslane, *Campanula poscharskyana, Claytonia virginica*. **Ground Cover Fruit** - Wild/alpine strawberries, dewberry, Japanese strawberry – raspberry, *Rubus tricolor, Rubus nutans*.

ROOT LEVEL - Onions, parsnip (which can be a good self-seeder), beetroot, Hamburg parsley, radish (black Spanish/Violet de Gournay), salsify, celeriac.

SELF-SEEDERS and ANNUALS - Rocket, (American) landcress, nasturtium, borage, radish, spinach, pick'n' pluck lettuces. Squashes and courgettes/zucchini are particularly productive, with many squashes being excellent winter foods that store well. Chilacayote is an amazing plant of this family for its large fruit and its long distance rambling habit - if you've got space!

FLOWERS - There is nothing more beautiful than a salad bowl laden with flowers: both delicious and beautiful are day lily, mallow, rose, chive, onion and garlic family flowers, borage and other herb flowers, milkweeds, yellow asphodel, nasturtium and calendula. Plants For A Future have a great website and book for more information on edible flowers.

Other Useful and Interesting Plants - Nettles are a wonderful green-juice plant, also the raw tips are tastey but have to be carefully picked with finger and thumb below the first sets of leaves, then rolled between finger and thumb - delicious and high in chlorophyll – useful as an early spring food source. And as a cooked food, nettles are probably as ecologically sound as you can get. Historically nettles have been an important fibre plant – and still are in some places in the world (see *Spirals of Abundance* for Nepalese nettle waistcoats, and more).

SUB-TROPICAL AND MEDITERRANEAN TYPE CLIMATES

The variety of plants and trees that can be grown is phenomenal once you get into warmer climates. The Australian book *Permaculture Plants* provides a lot of useful information including fast growing trees and shrubs that help improve, secure or rehabilitate the soil, as well as many drought tolerant species (e.g. tagasaste, albizia, leucaena). Robert Hart's book *Forest Gardening* has many useful suggestions for forest gardens in warmer climates, and includes more information on vegetables for these climates. *Introduction to Permaculture* also has a great deal of information on useful plants for these climates.

As with a temperate apple orchard it is relatively easy to transform a traditional orange grove (for example) to a much more diverse forest garden. Your choices include the following, some of which can provide crops for 6 to 8 months of the year if different varieties are selected, and/or different plants of the same variety are placed in subtly different micro-climates on site:

- Citrus: oranges, tangerines, grapefruit, lemons, ugli fruit and so on.
- Peaches, plums, pears, nectarines, kaki/sharon fruit/persimmon, many varieties of grapes, loquat, passion fruit, kiwi, azerole/edible hawthorn, apricots, figs, olives, pomegranite, prickly pear, mulberry, carob and so on.
- Avocados, cherimoyas/custard apple, jujube (Chinese date apple), papayas – hardier, non-commercial varieties can be tended through light frosts and will tolerate these once through their first few years. Mangos, banana and many other delicious fruit need to be frost free. Then there's pawpaw, sapodilla, white sapote, pepino, capuli, tamarillo, ice cream bean, various date palms, physallis and so on.
- Nuts: walnuts, almonds, pecans, chestnuts, pine nuts, etc.
- Many, many varieties of melon, including water melon.
- Cucumbers, numerous squashes, kiwano and a variety of trailing/climbing plants, including courgettes/zuchinni, chilacayote, and tomatoes.
- And a huge variety of perennial and annual vegetables, herbs and so on, including excellent seed producing plants such as sunflower.

At Ecoforest (southern Spain) we found rocket, spinach, chard, malva, fennel, various herbs, perennial broccoli, nasturtium, kale, wild and perennial onions, and others grow particularly well, with celery (for example) growing very happily under the orange trees.

- In tougher spots, drought tolerant soil improvers include tagasaste, leucaena, Ice cream bean, albizias, casaurinas – and many annual soil improving, nitrogen fixing plants such as alfalfa, chickpeas, peanuts, pigeon pea, clovers and other plants, including the so called 'wonder bean' from South America, the macuna bean.

The following table provides *indications* of seasons – exact seasons will vary according to variety, local climate and the micro-climate i.e. the positioning of different varieties of one type of fruit in sunny spots or shady spots will allow you to extend and vary the season of ripening. A range of salad plants can be easily grown below the fruit trees. With melons and watermelons it can be possible to start the season earlier where the plants are started in a conservatory, polytunnel or some other form of protection and then planted out when it is warm enough. Other vine fruits such as tomatoes and cucumbers can also be grown in this way, and with protection tomatoes or in frost free climates tomatoes can be grown all year round. Other fruits that can be grown include papaya and bananas where it is warm enough, olives, passionfruit, kiwi (does best with shade), sapote, lucuma, feijoa (pineapple guava), jujube (chinese date apple), guava (guayava), cactus fruit (prickly pear, chumbo), and many other types of fruit. Nuts that can be grown include almonds, pecans, walnuts, hazel nuts, chestnuts, and where it is warm enough macadamia and pistacio.

I thank the knowledgeable and inspiring Juan Ramos of Coin, Malaga (d.2003), a hugely experienced organic and permaculture grower in southern Spain (Mediterranean climate) for a great deal of the information in the table above.

FRUIT	January-March	April-June	July-September	Oct-December
Avocado	All year ...		(more scarce)	
Lemon	All year			
Orange		to June (July)		December start
Grapefruit	January-March	April-June		December start
Mandarin / Tangerine	January-March			Nov.-December
Chirimoya	March-April finish			October start
Loquat (Nispero)		April-May		
Apricot		Late April-May		
Strawberries		April-June		
Early Fig (Brevas)		May-June		
Cherry		May/June		
Plum		May-June		
Nectarine		April to	July	
Peach		April to	July	
Mulberry		May	to August	
Melons		May start		Nov. / Dec. finish
Watermelon		May start		Oct. / Nov.
Apple			June / July	to December
Pear			June / July	to December
Grape			June / July	to December
Fig			August-September	Oct-Nov. (Dec.)
Mango			September	to Nov/Dec.
Pomegranate			Sept. / Oct.	to December
Kaki (Persimmon)				Oct to Dec.

INDEX

There is no index to this book, as the Contents section is fairly extensive – and I hope through that you can find your way to any of the specifics you might want an Index for, albeit a little less directly. Apologies to anyone who is frustrated by this choice!

OTHER BOOKS BY STEVE CHARTER:

The Earth Dweller's Guide to Sustainability

This book is a unique exploration of the great challenges and opportunities we face. It is more readable, entertaining, stimulating and informative than the average book on sustainability that any 'student' of the issues (whether formal or informal) may have encountered. Exploring alternative views of sustainability, the progress we are making and the lack of it, the unique approach of this book takes the reader through a broad sustainability landscape, with depth, rigour and insight, from economics to culture to our patterns of thinking and values. This book provides practical and realistic guidance on the choice of paths we face, as individuals and as a culture, and will help any reader identify their practical next steps on the path. It's author is a sustainability practitioner, working with local government and business, as well as a teacher and has been involved in pioneering sustainability projects for more than 15 years.

(176 pages) Paperback, 2009

Available from http://www.lulu.com/content/4482469, £17.95 Download: £2.00

Sustainability, Consciousness and Climate Change

This book addresses the issue of the practical and pragmatic relationship between human consciousness, human sustainability and climate change. It focuses on and clarifies the direct relationship between the ways our consciousness functions, and malfunctions, and the fact that human cultures repeatedly create unsustainable ways of living, which result from unsustainable ways of thinking, which in turn result from unsustainable ways of perceiving our relationship to the world around us, other people and cultures and life on earth in general. This has hugely practical implications. This book argues that we have to utilise our consciousness and all the creative capacities that are associated with it to generate the most wise, positive and sustainable responses to the current state of humanity and the world – and that unless we recognize and act on the fact that our consciousness is the direct source of our problems, and solutions, we are entirely missing the point.

(88 pages) Paperback, 2009

Available from http://www.lulu.com/content/866695, £13.60 Download: £2.00

Sufficient Freedom (a novel)

This is work in progress ... Please feel free to encourage me to get it finished!

Steve has also written a number of guides to sustainable building.

The most important discovery in recorded history

RETURN TO THE BRAIN OF EDEN
Restoring the Connection between Neurochemistry and Consciousness

" It will be, it must be, taken very seriously in any discussion of human origins."Prof. Colin Groves (ANU)

"This is a startling book that makes us rethink the most fundamental issues of religion, psychology, and philosophy."Richard Heinberg (Post Carbon Institute)

"Left in the Dark offers a provocative and original answer to the most important question of our time." Linda Buzzell-Saltzman (IAE)

"WOW. Unless we do something radical it is bye bye" Prof. Michael A. Crawford. Director of the Institute of Brain Chemistry.

"This is an area that I know way too little about but from my uneducated take on all of this, it sure makes sense that we are paying a neuro-pathological price." Dr. Robert M Sapolsky. Professor of Neurology at Stanford University.

TONY WRIGHT AND GRAHAM GYNN
FOREWORD BY DENNIS J. McKENNA, PH.D.

The root cause of our obvious insanity and relentless capacity for self inflicted humanitarian and ecological catastrophe was staring us in the face, we were just too deluded to see it.

Return to the Brain of Eden
a mind blowing new book by Tony Wright

Tony Wright's amazing new discovery pieced together from established research into our evolutionary origins, the development of our brain and emergence of our mind answers 'The Question' that has eluded scientists and mystics alike since the dawn of civilisation. The implications are simply astounding and affect each and every one of us in every way.

Cause.
A simple diagnosis, the near total loss of a complex cocktail of design modifying compounds on the developmental and operating environment of the most chemically sensitive piece of kit we know.

Effect.
The unique molecular configuration and precise cellular architecture that effectively dictates our perception has changed out of all recognition. The development and function of our neural system is seriously retarded. Inevitably a mountain of data must already exist to support such a proposal, initial broad-spectrum reaction concurs, the evidence is overwhelming once you look for it.

email: info@kaleidos.org.uk
www.leftinthedark.org.uk